CHEF & DOCTOR
On The Run

by

Diane & Dr. Doug Clement

Sunflower Publications Ltd., Vancouver, B.C., Canada

Second printing October 1986

Sunflower Publications Ltd.,
1426 West 26th Avenue,
Vancouver, British Columbia,
Canada. V6H 2B4

Canadian Cataloguing in Publication Data

Clement, Diane 1936 —
Chef & doctor on the run

Includes index,
ISBN 0-920120-01-6

1. Nutrition. 2. Menus. 3. Cookery

I. Clement, Doug. II. Title.
TX731.C44 1986 641.5 C86-091483-6

Colour separations by Camart Studio Limited
Typeset by Benwell Atkins Ltd.
Printed and bound in Canada by Mitchell Press Ltd., Vancouver

Contents

Chapter One: The Doctor. A quick look at new dietary guidelines and recommended lifestyle changes for health and fitness. 2

Chapter Two: The Chef. Cooking with the new guidelines, hints and short-cuts, plus foods and kitchen equipment for the 80s. 8

Chapter Three: The Menus.

- Come for Lunch 19
- The Formal Picnic 23
- Exotic Tastes of the Middle East 29
- Mediterranean Feast 35
- Pasta Power 41
- In the Italian Tradition 46
- Light and Elegant 51
- Dinner on the Run 57
- The Contented Sole 62
- For Summer Entertaining 68
- Coast-to-Coast Celebration 74
- The Italian Connection 82
- California Pizzalina Party 86
- Fuel Foods 92
- The Flavours of India 99
- Sunday Brunch 104
- The Basics 108
- Comfort Foods 110

Chapter Four: An in-depth look at the whys and hows of the new dietary guidelines, plus a look at exercise 131

Index 146

To David, to mark the first 50 years

To Joel, our inspiration

To Ruth and Dianne for their endless support

ACKNOWLEDGEMENTS

Jack Bryan, food photography; Liz Bryan, copy editing and book design; Vicky Agar and Lynne Sawchuk, food analysis; Wise Owl Gift Tree, Vancouver, for exquisite table accessories (special thanks to Janet Anderson and her patient and capable staff, Nancy Scambler and Claudia Wakeman); Bill Donaldson, The Scale Shop, for the use of the scales on the cover; Barb Watts for her unique quality of always being there for advice and assistance; Glenys Morgan, Tools and Techniques, West Vancouver and Marilyn and her staff at Marilyn's in Delta for their enthusiasm when I teach at their cooking schools; Don and Marcelle McLean and Haik Gharibian, our friends, who opened their homes to us for food photography and also contributed recipes; students and friends for their encouragement to produce a cookbook stressing lighter cuisine and for taste-testing. We thank you all.

Introduction

Food is one of mankind's greatest pleasures and a central focus for entertaining friends and family. But how does it mesh with today's new lifestyle, a lifestyle very much concerned with health, nutrition and exercise? Will the food of the future sacrifice taste and visual appeal for nutritional and caloric values? Will the pleasures of the table be lost?

No, say Doug and Diane Clement. Healthy foods do not have to be boring. Neither will the lifestyle changes necessary for optimal health diminish the quality of life. This book reviews and recommends easy, but important lifestyle changes, including a shift to regular exercise. It discusses the main components of the food we eat and suggests areas of change, i.e. less fat, less sugar, less salt and more complex carbohydrates. But by far the largest part of the book consists of recipes, organized into sixteen complete menus for entertaining, that are consistent with the new principles yet amazingly tempting in both looks and taste. The easy-to-prepare dishes are fresh, innovative, stylish, satisfying — and best of all, delicious!

Diane Clement is literally a ''Chef on the Run''. She combines a lifetime involvement in sport with a 20-year background as a teacher of cooking and entertaining. She was an Olympic sprinter for Canada in 1956 and later the president of the Canadian Track and Field Association during the 1976 Olympic Games. She is still active as a manager of Canada's track and field team and keeps fit running 15 to 20 miles a week.

Dr. Doug Clement is co-director of the British Columbia Sports Medicine Centre and Associate Professor in the Faculty of Medicine at the University of British Columbia. He combines an active practice of sports medicine with research in the area of exercise-induced injuries and sports nutrition. He was an Olympic middle distance runner in 1952 and 1956 and remains active coaching Olympic runners. He was a sports physician for the Canadian Olympic team in 1984.

CHAPTER 1

The Doctor

Zap! A jolt of powerful electric current shot through my body. I jerked convulsively, my back arching upwards. It wasn't painful, exactly, but it sure as hell got my attention. This was pretty drastic treatment — and it had not worked! The EKG monitor beside the hospital bed showed my heart still beating wildly out of control, a condition known as atrial fibrillation which severely reduced its pumping action. I knew they would have to shock me again. The cardiologist approached to check the monitor and adjust the current.

Physicians are notoriously bad patients. We feel conspicuous, embarrassed. Here was I, a sports physician and a strong advocate of exercise and a healthy lifestyle, with an out-of-control cardiac arrhythmia! How could this happen to me? For a week I had experienced shortness of breath, dizziness and this wild irregular heart beat. Tests had uncovered no evidence of heart disease yet medications had failed to regulate the heart rhythm. I knew that defibrillation by electric shock was the only answer but knowing this did not decrease my apprehension. What if it failed again? I looked down at the paddles on my chest and crossed my fingers.

Zap! My body jerked even more convulsively but this time the EKG monitor showed a regular beat. My heart was back to normal. The strange fluttery feeling in my chest was gone, the crisis over. A little while later I got up and walked out of the hospital, as apparently healthy as ever.

This happened about ten years ago. I was in my mid-forties and actively fit; just about a month prior I had completed a marathon race. Exercise had always been a dominant part of my life, not only for myself but for my wife Diane and two children. I had met Diane at the 1956 Olympic Games in Melbourne in which we were both representing Canada, myself as a middle distance runner, Diane as a sprinter. Track and field activity remained an integral part of our lives, even after we were married and I entered the practice of general medicine in Richmond, B.C., a practice that, mainly because of my personal interest in sport, gradually shifted its emphasis towards sports medicine and problems related to exercise. We were both coaches, first at the community level, then for the Olympic Games and both kept very fit and active. In 1976 I joined the Department of Kinesiology at Simon Fraser University and later with my associate Dr. Jack Taunton was asked to form the inaugural Division of Sports Medicine at the University of British Columbia.

Throughout my whole career I had had no serious health problems beyond viral meningitis from which I had made a full recovery and a blow-out fracture of my left eye socket. This heart trouble must have a cause. I was fit, not overweight, I exercised regularly, did not smoke and drank alcohol only in moderation. Could it be the North American lifestyle? We are living in a period of tremendous affluence and tremendous technological change that affects all aspects of our lives, including our health. Most North Americans today suffer from a variety of conditions, many of which are caused by affluence. For men, the leading causes of death in the middle years are heart disease, lung cancer, motor vehicle accidents, cirrhosis of the liver, cerebral vascular disease (strokes), various forms of intestinal and stomach cancer and other diseases. Could my heart problems be related to my lifestyle? I decided to look into it.

It is chiefly because of the spirally rising costs of health care that the governments of both the US and Canada have taken that old saying to heart: "prevention is better than cure" and are trying to effect changes in certain aspects of lifestyle believed to be detrimental to health. Studies have been taking place for years and by the late 1970s, independent health organizations in both countries had come up with almost identical recommendations which can be summarized as follows:

1. It is better to be slim than fat.
2. It is better not to smoke cigarettes.
3. Exercise and fitness are better than sedentary living.
4. Alcohol is a danger to health and is a particular risk when driving an automobile.
5. Tranquillity is better than excess stress.
6. Excessive use of medication, particularly of mood-modifying drugs, is to be avoided.
7. Air and water should be polluted as little as possible.

Diet

In 1977, a committee established in the United States on Nutrition and Human Needs (the McGovern Committee) showed the average North American diet to be 42% fat, 12% protein and 46% carbohydrate. The fat intake consisted of 16% saturated, 19% mono-unsaturated and 7% polyunsaturated. Carbohydrate consumption broke down into 22% complex carbohydrate, 6% simple sugar and 18% processed sugar.

The McGovern Committee established new dietary goals which would increase the nation's level of fitness. These are:

Fat: Decrease consumption to 30%, with equal quantities of saturated, mono-unsaturated and polyunsaturated;

Protein: Keep constant at 12%.

Carbohydrate: Increase to 58%, only 10% of which should be in the form of processed sugar.

This may seem like drastic change but only as regards recent eating habits. These recommendations are almost exactly in line with the average diet in 1910. In one sense at least, those were the good old days. Today, three out of every five calories in the North American diet come from fats and refined sugars. Two out of every five people on this continent are obese.

The recommendations of the Human Nutrition Centre are as follows:

1. Eat a variety of foods.
2. Maintain ideal weight.
3. Avoid fat, both saturated and cholesterol.
4. Avoid sodium and salt
5. Avoid sugar.
6. Eat food with starch and fibre.
7. Drink only moderate amounts of alcohol.

When I first read these recommendations and compared them to my own diet, I realized that my food intake could be a contributory factor in my heart condition. Our house was known to be a centre for good eating. During my internship in San Francisco Diane had become intensely interested in cooking and foods, an interest that has if anything accelerated over the years. Back in Vancouver she started a cooking school and in recent years, as Chef on the Run, she has written a couple of best-selling cookbooks. I was becoming known as the husband of the Chef on the Run, and I enjoyed the notoriety. All this meant, however, that at home we ate very well indeed, as most of the rest of North Americans still do. What would it take in our lives to adjust our diet to the new regime of low fat, low salt, low sugar, high carbohydrate? And would this alleviate my heart problem?

I thought about it a lot, read many books and papers on nutrition and eventually decided to try. Gradually over the past 10 years, and with Diane's full support, we have adopted the new dietary regime. It was not difficult to do, nor do we feel deprived. The first thing to be reduced in our family was fat: we switched to skim milk and stopped using butter and margarine on our bread. Next we gave up sugar in tea and coffee. Then, because it was considered that caffeine as a heart stimulant might be the critical trigger of my atrial fibrillation problems, I switched over to decaffeinated coffee and gave up tea and later chocolate altogether. Soft drinks, particularly colas which contain caffeine, were also dropped. None of these changes took place all at once and sometimes I confess I would slip back into the old ways; but my heart would start acting up again and my experience with electric-shock treatment was certainly reason enough to stay on the new course.

One of the more recent things to go was ice cream, a substantial source of fat and sugar. It's not that an occasional scoop would hurt but I'm afraid I have a tendency, once I start on ice cream, to go on a binge and eat a whole quart. It's the same with cookies, particularly chocolate chip cookies. In the last three or four years I have avoided the temptation altogether.

Slowly, too, we have moved away from the consumption of red meats and increased our use of fish, seafood and poultry. We always take off the poultry skin, since this is where most of the fat resides, and avoid frying our foods. We stopped using salt at the table and Diane has cut it back in cooking. The new regime has meant a kitchen revolution for Diane who was famous for her cream sauces and rich foods, and the transformation has not been without emotional trauma. But in this book Diane has shown that eating right can also be delicious and every bit as adventurous and satisfying. More, we feel better; we're slimmer, we have more energy.

The whole area of nutrition is a complex one and as a discipline is still in its formative stages. There is a great deal of confusion and conflicting opinion regarding food and its effect on health, and many advocates of the crash diet. But any approach to change must look at lifestyle; food is only part of the totality of habits that we lock under the term ''lifestyle''. Exercise, the use of drugs and alcohol, cigarette smoking, the amount of stress in our lives, all contribute to our general health. We are not only what we eat, but what we do.

Because this is essentially a cookbook, the emphasis here is on nutrition. The ideas I put foward are not my own but a distillation of several sources. They represent, however, only an intelligent best guess because so far there is no direct proof that nutrition can affect disease processes, though I consider it highly likely. Let's look at the new dietary and lifestyle goals and how best to achieve them.

A Health & Fitness Diet for the 80s

Less Total Fat. Reduce from 42% of daily calorie intake to 30%
Why? To reduce risk of breast, colon and prostate cancers, and heart disease, strokes and gallstones.
How? Drastically cut down on butter and margarine, mayonnaise, creams, oil, visible animal fat, rich pastries and desserts, fried foods, etc. Choose fish and poultry over red meat.

Choose Polyunsaturated Fats over Saturated
Why? Polyunsaturated fats may decrease blood cholesterol levels.
How? Use vegetable oils instead of butter and lard; decrease use of animal fats (meat, cream, butter), cheese; avoid hard vegetable fats such as coconut oil, cocoa butter.

Cut Back Refined Sugar from 18% to 10%
Why? Refined sugar provides a high concentration of calories, easily converted to fat; excess sugar promotes tooth decay.
How? Give up candy bars, cakes, pies, cookies, sugar in tea and coffee and sugar-sweetened soft drinks; reduce amount of sugar in home baking; avoid processed foods high in sugar.

Increase daily intake of starches and fibre from 46% to 58%

Why? To replace calories lost from decreased fat intake; to provide bulk, minerals and vitamins. Increased fibre intake may reduce cancer of the colon and intestines.
How? Eat more whole grains, breads, cereals, pasta, potatoes, beans, fresh fruits and vegetables.

Cut Down Salt Intake to 5 grams a day
Why? Salt intake is linked to high blood pressure.
How? Add no salt at the table; reduce or eliminate salt in cooking and food preparation.

Keep Protein Consumption at 12%
Why? Bodies need protein. Eight of the essential amino acids must be supplied from food intake. An average 160 lb man needs 57 grams of protein a day. Too much protein can stress the liver (which breaks down amino acids into carbohydrate and nitrogen) and kidneys, and may increase the loss of calcium from the body (which can lead to osteoporosis (brittle bones) and fractures).

How? The best source of protein is derived from animals: milk, eggs, cheese, meat, fish, poultry. But these can also be high in fat. Choose wisely and watch portion size. Shift protein intake from animal to vegetable sources, remembering that vegetable proteins are incomplete and must be paired, i.e. legumes plus grain; legumes plus seeds.

Lifestyle Changes

Give up Smoking
Why? Smoking definitely increases the risk of lung cancer and other lung diseases, plus diseases of coronary arteries.

Moderate Alcohol Use
Why? Heavy use causes high blood pressure, weakens heart muscles and adversely affects brain, liver and gastro-intestinal tract. There is a high incidence of death and injury from drunken driving. **Moderate** use of alcohol (1 to 2 drinks a day) decreases risk of coronary artery disease.

Reduce Caffeine Intake
Why? Caffeine is addictive, increases heart rate and metabolism and stimulates kidneys.

Decrease Stress
Why? Stress increases risk of heart disease.

Increase Physical Activity
Why? To keep cardio-vascular system healthy and body young. Help burn off excess calories and maintain ideal body weight.

(For a more detailed look at today's healthier approach to food and more discussion of lifestyle changes, please turn to Chapter 4)

CHAPTER 2

The Chef

Even after the shock of having Doug rushed to hospital with a heart problem, it took me some time to realize that our eating habits must change. Doug had started by himself, cutting down on sugar and fats but I continued cooking with heavy cream, chocolate and butter, not just for my family, but with my cooking students.

''What are you trying to do? Kill everyone?'' Doug used to say as he watched me loading on the sugar and the egg yolks. At first I thought he was joking. But he kept after me, and I finally faced the fact that the good food I had been serving my friends and family for years was not always good for them. So I changed to a new healthier style of cooking, using less fat, less sugar and less salt. It was for me a revolution. But I could see I was not alone. It was beginning to happen all over the western world as part of the increasing emphasis on fitness: people wanted food that was nutritionally well balanced, energy boosting, would not make them fat, and also tasted good. The ''nature'' foods of the 70s had failed in this regard because they were dull and unappetizing. Today's foods are light and fresh and above all, delicious.

When they saw that ''the new diet'' was *in fact* delicious, my family and friends urged me to put together a cookbook reflecting the new approach. This was a challenge indeed, particularly as all the menus had to meet the exacting taste and presentation standards of my two previous Chef on the Run cookbooks. Any recipe, no matter how nutritious, had to taste and look good, or it was not included. I used some egg yolks, sugar, butter and oil, but only in small quantities when I felt they were needed to enhance flavour or texture. A little goes a long way to produce excellent results.

Cooks will discover that this healthier approach to food will change their shopping habits: they will shop much more frequently for the freshest products; but it will cut down on the time they spend in the kichen; preparation and cooking times are reduced. (I usually have a complete meal on the table within 30 to 45 minutes.) However, I have designed the menus in this book so that, if you are entertaining, much of the preparation can be done ahead of time.

Helpful Hints

Remember, your everyday meals should be as healthy as possible and often this will not mean that drastic changes are required. Just keep in mind the goals of low fat, low sugar, low salt and high complex carbohydrate (starches). Here are some simple pointers to a new direction in eating:

* Serve only moderate amounts of food and fewer dishes per meal. Rely on poultry, veal and fish rather than red meats and serve very small portions of these, trimming off all visible fat and removing poultry skin. Remember, only 12% of your daily food intake should consist of protein, and that protein is also found in cheese, eggs, whole grains and other foods besides meat and fish. Serve larger portions of vegetables, fruits and grains.
* Contrast flavours, colours and textures. Food should always be tempting to the eye as well as to the palate. For best flavour, serve hot food on warm plates, cold food on chilled plates.
* To keep calories down when entertaining, eliminate the appetizer course and go straight to the soup or salad. Save the rich cream pies and cakes for a special occasion; your guests will be just as pleased with a fresh fruit dessert.
* Steam or lightly saute vegetables for best taste, appearance and goodness. When sauteeing, use a non-stick pan sprayed with a little vegetable oil (fill a plant mister with oil or buy a commercial spray such as Pam). The vegetables can also be partly covered with parchment or a lid to make them "sweat" moisture which will prevent them from scorching.
* If you always serve good quality fresh bread, you will not need butter or margarine. Remember that 1 tablespoon (15 mL) of butter equals 100 calories.
* Thicken sauces with a little cornstarch or arrowroot mixed with wine or stock. You'll need less arrowroot than flour and will not need to use butter.
* Bouillon cubes are convenient but they contain large amounts of salt for preservation. Homemade stock is not only less salty, it tastes better.
* Don't hesitate to use a little wine in your cooking. Most of the alcohol (calories) evaporates in the cooking process but the flavour remains.
* To reduce fats in soups and stews, cook them ahead of time, then chill and skim off the fat solids before you reheat and serve.

* Substitute skim milk for whole milk. When I first started to buy skim milk, my children said, "Oh Mom! It's gross!" but now they are used to it they find even 2% milk too rich. On occasion I will use 2% milk in some sauces that normally call for butter. It improves the texture. Exchanging skim milk for whole milk will mean a saving of 72 calories and about 8 grams of fat for each 8-ounce (250 mL) glass. If you drink three glasses of milk a day, this adds up to a saving of 216 calories and 24 grams of fat.

* Use low fat or 2% yogurt instead of sour cream or whipping cream for sauces and dressings. One cup (250 mL) of low fat yogurt equals 122 calories; 1 cup of sour cream equals 494 calories. Mixing yogurt with a teaspoon (5 mL) or so of cornstarch before adding it to a sauce will prevent curdling. For creamier sauces, I sometimes use half low-fat yogurt and half regular yogurt. Yogurt can also be made thicker by straining off the whey in a cheesecloth-lined collander.

* Substitute whole wheat flour for all or part of the white flour called for in a recipe and choose recipes for whole-grain breads and muffins, cutting down on the sugar required. It's amazing how little sugar you need in a muffin, for example, particularly if it's stuffed with raisins or other dried fruits. For moist muffins and coffeecakes, use buttermilk instead of regular milk. Buttermilk, the whey left over from the butter-making process, is nutritious and naturally low-fat.

* When a recipe calls for eggs, substitute 1 egg plus 1 egg white for every 2 whole eggs to reduce cholesterol intake.

* Remember one basic rule: you can't eat it if you don't have it. In other words, don't keep in the house such tempting things as rich cakes, cookies, chocolate, ice cream, candies, high fat cheeses, potato chips, nuts and other nibblies. Instead keep on hand plenty of fresh fruits and vegetables, unbuttered popcorn for snacks, and supplies of bran and whole-grain muffins and breads. You'll be surprised at how soon you adapt to the new regime. And how much healthier you feel.

* Start every day with a good breakfast, but give up bacon and eggs. In our house we start with fruit juice, hot or cold whole-grain cereal (porridge in winter with skim milk and fresh or dried fruit instead of brown sugar) or a healthy muffin (no butter).

* Low-cal mayonnaise is a fine substitute for butter on sandwiches, or use small amounts of polyunsaturated margarine. Sandwich fillings can be treacherous: don't buy bologna or other packaged meats or processed cheeses. Rely instead on lean meats, sprouts, tomatoes, cucumber, lettuce or water-packed tuna.

* Fructose is actually a natural sugar found in fruits and honey. It's sweeter than most sugar so less is required; substitute approximately 1/2 teaspoon fructose for 1 teaspoon sugar in recipes. It can be found in most health food sections.

Star Foods of the 80s

Food is like fashion: styles and trends come and go but a few classics are popular for generations. Like fashion, food should be dramatic, enticing and seductive. It should always bring pleasure. Food of the 80s certainly has no excuse being dull. There is far more variety available today than ever before — pasta in a dozen shapes and flavours; fresh fish and seafoods, exotic fruits and vegetables, whole grains, cheeses and yogurts, ethnic and regional specialties, fresh herbs and exotic spices. The local food market has become an international bazaar, its deli counters a visual feast from around the world. Here are some of my favourite Foods of the 80s.

Chevre Cheese

Made from the milk of goats, this smooth and creamy cheese is much lower in butterfat compared to other hard cheeses (20% butterfat, as against up to 40% butterfat for Cheddar, Brie and Camembert). Always popular in its native France, it was introduced to North America by California chefs (who traditionally take the lead when it comes to food trends and styles). Today chevre is made commercially in both the U.S. and Canada and you'll find the local product milder than the European. Chevre is excellent for making sauces as it does not curdle when heated. It melts easily, too.

Parmesan Cheese

This familiar Italian cheese is also relatively low in fat content, 20 to 25%, and since fresh Parmesan is robust in flavour, less of it is needed. Avoid tinned, pre-grated Parmesan with its additives and buy fresh hunks from your local deli. My first choice would be Parmigiano Reggiano, from Italy's Parma region. One of the finest cheeses in the world, it is aged in Italy for a minimum of 18 months before it can be sold. It is made by hand, is yellow in colour and should crumble easily. For best flavour, grate your own Parmesan at the last moment and don't discard the hard heel — it's marvellous added to soup or tomato sauce. Just throw it in while the soup or sauce is cooking, then remove just before you serve. It adds a fine flavour. (Keep the heels in the freezer until you need them.)

Ricotta

Another cheese low in fat, ricotta is made from whey, the watery milk residue left from the cheese-making process. It is ideal for lasagne, stuffing noodles and desserts. Use it to replace creamed cottage cheese or cream cheese.

Mozzarella Cheese

Substitute part-skim mozzarella cheese (often as low as 15% butterfat) for toppings or sauces.

Cottage Cheese

Use low-fat cottage cheese (2% butterfat) instead of creamed (4%).

Oils

Oil, like all fat, should be used sparingly. For sauteeing meats and vegetables, I use a non-stick frypan lightly sprayed with a vegetable oil spray. The best oils to use in cooking are the polyunsaturated kinds such as safflower or sunflower. Use olive oil, which is a mono-unsaturated oil, sparingly. I keep my olive oil in the refrigerator as its shelf life is very short. **Extra virgin olive oil** (from the first pressing of the olives) is light and delicate in flavour, worth the extra cost. For salads, try **Walnut Oil**, also a polyunsaturate, and with a rich flavour. **Dark Sesame Oil** is slightly thick and has a full-bodied flavour. Made from roasted sesame seeds and light brown in colour, it is used more for seasoning than for cooking because it burns easily. It is popular in Chinese dishes.

To accentuate vegetables or pasta sauce, I use a home-made **Red Pepper Oil**. Bring one cup (250 mL) of safflower oil to a boil, remove from heat and add 1 tablespoon (15 mL) red pepper flakes. Leave to steep for about 30 minutes. Strain oil and store in refrigerator for up to a month or so. Use only a little: its flavour is intense.

Vinegars

Many exotic vinegars are making their appearance on today's grocery shelves. Fruit vinegars such as raspberry and blueberry are popular in salads, for marinating chicken and with fresh fruit. You can easily make you own. When fresh fruits such as strawberries, peaches or apples are past their prime, slice them thinly and add to white vinegar. Store in the refrigerator for a day or so, then strain and use. Herb vinegars such as tarragon or basil also add an intriguing dimension to salads and marinades. Always buy a good quality vinegar. An inferior product can ruin a dish.

My favourite vinegar is **Balsamic**. It is easily identified by its dark brown colour. Unlike other vinegars made from grape juice, this one is made from the unfermented must of white Trebbiano grapes that has been boiled down to a sweet concentrate and it must by law be aged for at least ten years in wooden casks before it can be sold. As a result, it is more expensive than other vinegars but its flavour is intense and you will need to use less of it. It is highly aromatic. Its marvellous flavour arouses the taste buds when sprinkled on grilled meats, fish or vegetables. And it's sheer delight sprinkled lightly on fresh strawberries. Yes, balsamic vinegar is definitely here to stay.

Rice Vinegar made from fermented rice is mild and slightly sweet, used often in Chinese cooking. **Sherry Vinegar** is also popular in Chinese cooking and makes a delicate fruit-flavoured salad dressing, too.

Vegetables

Yes, there are fashions in vegetables, too. Some of these "newest sensations" have been around a long time. **Bell Peppers**, the red and yellow varieties, are definitely the hottest rage. I personally find green peppers hard to digest so I prefer to use the red pepper (which is actually a ripe green pepper) because it is sweeter and more delicate in flavour. Yellow peppers are also mild and their colour is vibrant. Together, red and green peppers add excitement and great taste to any dish. Serve them raw or briefly sauteed, and store them like mushrooms: in a brown paper bag in a refrigerator vegetable bin. Try peppers on the barbecue. Leave them whole, rub with a little vegetable oil and place on the grill, turning often, for about 8 to 10 minutes. The skins will turn black. Put them in a paper bag for a few minutes, then peel, seed and slice. They're fabulous!

Bok Choy, or Chinese cabbage, used to be found only in Chinese markets and in Oriental stir-fry dishes. Today it's popular for salads. Cut off the root ends and pull off the stalks. Discard any tough leaves and the hard ribs and cut into strips.

Fennel, which looks a bit like a bulbous celery plant, is known in Europe as anise or finochio. It has a faint licorice flavour. Its feathery leaves make ideal garnish and the root can be sliced for soups, stews, braised as a side dish or eaten raw as appetizers or in salads.

Leeks are back in favour. Like giant green onions, they have flat green leaves and thick white stalks. The green tops are usually discarded and only the white portion used. They are great braised and make interesting additions to soups and sauces. Choose thin ones: the thick stems tend to be tough.

Lettuce Greens. There are some newcomers here, such as radicchio, in addition to the old favourites, romaine, leafy lettuce and spinach. Radicchio is a small, round and deep red Italian lettuce. Its delicate leaves have a piquant, almost bitter taste which seem to complement other greens, and its vibrant colour lights up any salad. It's mostly imported from Northern Italy so it's not always easy to find and it is expensive. (But one tiny head will be enough for six or eight people.) However, it is now being grown locally, so its price and availability should improve. It complements chevre cheese beautifully.

Mushrooms

In addition to the regular brown or white button mushrooms, several interesting wild varieties are making their appearance in produce markets. **Shiitake** or Black Forest mushrooms have always been common in Oriental cuisine but today are gaining in popularity for all dishes. They are dark brown, umbrella-shaped and have a beautifully subtle taste and sensual texture. Enjoy them on their own, sauteed quickly for a few seconds in a hint of butter. I find the stems a bit tough so I remove them and freeze them for adding later to soups. Shiitake mushrooms are now being grown commercially in a few places.

Chanterelles are reddish orange in colour and shaped like a frilly- edged cup. Steam them lightly or saute with a bit of butter and pepper. **Oyster mushrooms** are delicate grey and can be used in much the same way as the chanterelles. Both add a unique flavour to sauces or are exquisite on their own.

Perhaps the prince of all the mushrooms is the **Morel** which grows in the spring. It has a tall cone-shaped cap that is pock-marked like a sponge. Its rich flavour is unforgettable. Fresh morels are difficult to find (they have so far not been cultivated) and even more difficult to clean. I use dried morels which can be found in specialty shops. Soak the dried mushrooms in stock or water for an hour or so until they are soft, then drain and saute quickly. (Save the soaking stock for soups or sauces.)

Dijon Mustard. As anyone who has read my other books knows, I put Dijon mustard in everything but dessert. This specialty from the capital of Burgundy gives a lift to salad dressings, sauces, stews and meat coatings. Many delis are now making their own mustard varieties using herbs, spices and honey. Try them out. Store these and all mustards once they are opened in the refrigerator.

Pine Nuts (Pignoli). Most nuts are high in cholesterol and should be used sparingly. For special dishes I enjoy the small and creamy pine nuts, the fruit of a variety of pine tree. Round and sweet, they are most frequently used in Greek, Spanish and Italian dishes. Be sure they are fresh when you buy them: they go stale quickly. Keep them in the freezer. I like to toast them before using as this brings out their flavour. Just brown them on a tray in a medium oven for about five minutes or until they turn golden.

Shallots. I prefer these to onions because they are more easily digested. They look like miniature brown-skinned onions and in flavour are a cross between onions and garlic, but sweeter. Use them in everything that calls for onions and garlic.

Rice

As Reay Tannahill discovered in her excellent book ''Food in History'', rice is the principal food of 60% of the world's population. There are about 7,000 known strains of rice, all of which can be divided into long, medium and short grain. Long grain is the preferred variety for main dishes. Short grain rice which contains more starch is better for puddings or moulded dished. **Arborio** is an Italian short grain rice with the clinging quality necessary for the smooth consistency of properly cooked risotto.

Brown Rice is simply rice that has undergone less milling. The milling process in white rice removes the outer hull and all the bran layers, while in brown rice, only some of the bran layers are removed. It is the bran layers that give brown rice its characteristic colour, its pleasant nut-like taste and crunchy texture. Brown rice, which can be long or short grain, is definitely more nutritious than white, containing more protein, calcium, phosphorus, potassium, niacin and vitamin E. Because of its bran layer, it takes longer to cook and should be started in cold water. It will never be as tender as white rice. To keep it fresh, store brown rice in the refrigerator. Don't wash it before cooking as this will remove some of the nutrients.

Basmati Rice, one of the world's finest long grain varieties, is grown in the foothills of the Himalayas. It is popular in Indian cooking and has a fine aroma and intriguing taste. I like to use it with chicken. **Wild Rice** isn't really rice at all. It's the seed of certain types of aquatic grasses that grow in shallow ponds or marshes, particularly in the northern prairie provinces. It must be harvested by hand and because of this it is always expensive. However, a little goes a long way — it triples in volume when cooked. High in fibre and low in fat, wild rice has about 100 calories per half-cup (125mL) serving, 4 grams of protein, 0.4 grams of fat, 20 grams of carbohydrate and 60 mg of potassium.

Sun-Dried Tomatoes. These have recently become popular not for Italian dishes alone but for nearly everything, a particularly welcome addition to salads, sauces and stews. Dried in the sun then preserved in olive oil, they are available at most Italian specialty stores. They have a concentrated flavour and although expensive, you need to use very little for the effect and flavour you need. I slice or cube them small and use a little of their oil for sauteeing vegetables or for a salad dressing. When you buy them, ask to have a little extra oil and store them in an airtight container in the refrigerator.

Japanese Cuisine. When we dine out, we particularly enjoy Japanese cuisine. It's low in fat, light and fresh and the presentation is dramatic.

Herbs and Spices

Because the healthier style of cooking omits the use of salt, herbs and spices are important to boost the flavours of food. Dried herbs and spices will keep their flavour only for about 6 months, then they start to deteriorate. Put dates on your jars and check for flavour when they start to get old. You may have to use more for the same effect. If there is little aroma left, throw it out and buy new stock — in small quantities. Fresh herbs are always preferable and many greengrocers can now supply them, though usually only on a seasonal basis. Several of them can be grown indoors year-round so it's a good idea to plant your own kitchen herb garden. Use three times the amount of fresh herbs as dried — and be prepared for a totally different flavour. Again, here are the current favourites:

Basil is one herb that in the larger centres is available fresh year-round and is exceptionally easy to grow at home. Basil gives a unique flavour to Italian pasta sauces and is a perfect match for fresh ripe tomatoes and a good olive oil.

Cumin is a member of the parsley family and it has a slightly bitter taste. Only the seeds, which resemble those of caraway in both looks and flavour, are used in cooking. It is a basic spice for curries and Middle Eastern cuisine.

Cilantro or Chinese Parsley is a member of the coriander family. Its flat green leaves have a distinctive aroma and taste and should be used sparingly. It is often used in Chinese and Mexican dishes and makes an elegant garnish.

Dill is grown in most home vegetable gardens because it is a staple for pickle making. It is available fresh most of the year in produce markets. It adds a distinctive flavour to soups and salad dressings and many ethnic dishes. Its feathery leaves make a pretty garnish.

Fennel. Because of its sweet licorice flavour, this vegetable is also used as a herb. It's excellent with fish and chopped in soups and salads. Both the stalks and feathery leaves are used.

Garlic is not really a herb or a spice but because of its intense flavour it is usually considered as such. It is actually a member of the lily family. You either hate its pungency or you love it. I never ate it when I was young until I read somewhere that the ancients spoke of it as a magical energy food. I've eaten it ever since although I don't think there's anything magic about it, except its flavour. Fresh garlic is available everywhere, year-round. So why bother with the dried stuff? Be careful not to burn garlic when you saute it; this will give it a bitter taste. If you do burn it, even slightly, throw it out, wash the pan and start over. It's a good idea to saute onion and garlic together so that the onion juices will prevent scorching.

Ginger Root is a light brown knobby root with a powerful ginger flavour. To use, scrape off the peel with a sharp knife then grate or finely chop. For short storage, keep in the refrigerator. Freeze for longer periods and just cut off what you need while it is still frozen — you only need tiny amounts. To preserve the ginger, peel and slice thinly and store in the refrigerator in a glass jar with just enough medium dry sherry to cover. This will keep for about three months.

Turmeric contains a bright yellow dye that gives its distinctive colour to curries and other Far Eastern dishes. It can also be used in place of saffron to give colour to food, although it has a slightly bitter taste. It is the root of a member of the ginger family and it is usually only available in powdered form.

Storing Fresh Herbs is not a problem if you grow your own, you simply pick what you need. If you buy bunches of herbs however, they will keep for up to a week in the refrigerator. Some such as parsley can be treated like flowers, put into a glass of water, covered with a plastic bag and refrigerated. Others, such as basil, thyme, rosemary, etc. should be patted dry, wrapped in paper towels and stored in plastic bags in the vegetable compartment. Fresh herbs can also be chopped finely and frozen in ice-cube trays. Put about 1 tablespoon (15 mL) in each cube, fill with water to cover and freeze. Store frozen herb cubes in a plastic bag and add to soups and stews as required. The herbs might turn dark but they will keep their fresh flavour for up to six months.

Some Facts on Fish

Growing up in the Maritimes and now living on the West Coast, I tend to take fresh fish for granted. Luckily, frozen fish and seafood are now available across the country. When choosing frozen products, make sure the container has no leaks and very few crystals. If possible, buy flash-frozen, which means the fish is frozen on the boat immediately after it is caught for best flavour. Frozen fish will keep up to two months in the freezer but once thawed should be cooked immediately.

When choosing fresh fish, look for moist, shiny skin with no grey around the edges. When you press down on the fish, the flesh should spring back. Don't buy it if it has a ''fishy'' smell; fresh fish is almost odorless.

Store fresh fish in the coolest part of the refrigerator, lightly covered with waxed paper. Use within two days.

Cook fish lightly. When it ''flakes'' it may be too dry. Instead, look for colour changes. Fish is done when it turns from translucent to opaque and just begins to fall apart around the edges. For baking, allow about 10 minutes per inch of thickness in a 425 degree oven or grill about five minutes on each side.

Nutrition Analysis Notes

Each recipe has been analysed for number of calories per serving, based on the largest number of recommended servings. Optional ingredients have been omitted from the calculations. In addition, single servings for the complete menu have been analysed for the percentage of calories derived from protein, carbohydrate and fat, as well as the total amounts of sodium and cholesterol in each serving. You'll see that these do not, in most cases, meet the recommended percentages of 12 % protein, 30% fat and 58% carbohydrate, but remember that the menus represent the main meal of the day, a meal that is most likely to contain a higher proportion of protein and fat. What you eat for breakfast, lunch and snacks will obviously influence the total daily percentages.

From a nutritional point of view, target percentages should be worked out over a two or three day period; this allows for single meal fluctuations — and even the occasional splurge.

CHAPTER 3

The Recipes

Come for Lunch

Spritzer

Chilled Melon Soup

Oriental Chicken Salad

Wholewheat or Sourdough Bread

Banana Ice with Raspberry Puree

Luncheon fare is traditionally light, satisfying without being filling. This lunch menu is ideal for summer entertaining since all but the dessert can be made in advance — and the dessert can be made in three seconds flat! It starts with a refreshing cold melon soup, made with two varieties of melon, green and orange, poured together in a yin-yang design. The crisp tangy salad has a definite Oriental flavour and can be served either on a bed of curly-leaf lettuce or in a hollowed-out loaf of bread. The dessert, which must be whipped up at the last minute, is fun, refreshing and healthy.

Analysis

Serves 4
668 calories per serving
Protein: 19%
Fat: 19%
Carbohydrate: 62%
Sodium: 1247 mg
Cholesterol: 45 mg

(Photo following page 28)

Spritzer

(65 calories per serving)

For this, use half sparkling mineral water and half dry white wine, served over lots of ice cubes with a good twist of lemon or lime.

Add an ounce or two of raspberry or strawberry puree for a fruit spritzer.

Chilled Melon Soup

(125 calories per serving)

Melons are one of the healthiest, most nutritious of fruits and low in calories, too. Half a melon contains only 60 calories. This soup must be served well chilled. Serves 4.

1 large, ripe honeydew melon, chilled
2 teaspoons (10 mL) fresh lime juice
grated zest of 1 lime
1 teaspoon (5 mL) chopped fresh mint
(or good pinch of dried mint)
1 large ripe cantaloupe melon, chilled
1 teaspoon (5 mL) lemon juice
grated zest of half a lemon
fresh mint sprigs for garnish

The day ahead or on the morning of serving, peel and seed both melons and cut into large cubes. Combine honeydew with lime juice, zest and mint and blend well. Pour into small pitcher and refrigerate. Repeat with the cantaloupe, lemon juice and zest, and refrigerate in a separate pitcher.

To serve, set out four individual-size clear glass bowls. Pour small, equal amounts of the two melon mixtures simultaneously into each bowl and garnish with a mint sprig. Additional chopped melon can be added to the soup, if desired.

Oriental Chicken Salad

(273 calories per serving)

This complete meal salad is a favourite choice when athletes drop in for lunch after a workout and for weekend guests. Great for picnics and for stuffing in pita pockets, it can be made the day ahead of serving. Serves 6.

2 cups (500mL) fresh snow pea pods (or green beans)
3 green onions, chopped
2 cups (500 mL) cooked chicken breast, sliced into strips
1 cup (250 mL) red and/or yellow pepper, in julienne strips
1/2 cup (125 mL) coarsely chopped pecans, toasted almonds or cashews
2 cups (500 mL) fresh bean sprouts
(preferably a mixture of lentil, mung and chick peas)
2 tomatoes, peeled, seeded and cubed
1 to 2 large heads romaine or leafy lettuce, cleaned

Cut the tips off the pea pods or beans and blanch in boiling water for about 30 seconds. Chill immediately in ice water and pat dry. Combine all the ingredients except for lettuce leaves and toss with enough dressing to coat. Chill several hours or overnight. To serve: hollow out a large long or round loaf of wholewheat or sourdough bread and fill with the chicken mixture. Or pile chicken salad on a large platter lined with the leafy lettuce and serve the bread separately. Pass extra dressing.

Dressing

Serves 16.

1/4 cup (60 ml) vegetable oil
1/4 cup (60 mL) lemon juice
grated zest of 1 lemon
2 tablespoons plus 1 teaspoon (35 mL) low-sodium soy sauce
1/2 teaspoon (2 mL) powdered ginger
1 clove garlic, crushed
4 tablespoons (60 mL) light mayonnaise
4 tablespoons (60 mL) low fat yogurt, strained
Pepper to taste

Blend well and store, covered, in refrigerator. This can be made a day or two ahead.

Banana Ice with Raspberry Puree

(133 calories per serving)

This intriguing dish has everyone guessing the ingredients and everyone scooping up the last delicious mouthful. Smooth and creamy, yet low cal, I call it my ''energy revitalizer''. For a change, serve it with a blueberry or strawberry puree. Serves 4 to 6.

On the day of serving, peel four or five bananas, dip them in lemon juice and freeze. Bananas should be fully ripe but not dark. Allow four to five hours for them to freeze firm.

Just before serving, cut frozen bananas into chunks and zap in food processor or blender with about 3 tablespoons (45 mL) of plain, orange or pineapple yogurt and whirl until blended smooth. Place about 2 tablespoons (30 mL) of raspberry puree on each serving plate, place a scoop of banana ice on top and garnish with fresh raspberries if available and a sprig of fresh mint.

Note: Serve this fast. The banana ice, which has the consistency of soft ice-cream, will quickly melt. It cannot be made and frozen ahead.

Raspberry Puree

Puree 2 cups (500 mL) of fresh or frozen unsweetened raspberries, then strain in fine mesh strainer. This can be made ahead and frozen (allow to thaw overnight) or kept in the refrigerator for several days.

The Formal Picnic

Turkey or Chicken Breast
with Spinach Stuffing
and Curry Sauce

Salad Primavera

Oriental Noodle Salad

Wholewheat Sourdough Bread
and Assorted Baguettes

Fresh Fruit
with Sauce of the Happy Spices

Oatmeal Hearts

The Victorians were famous for their elegant gargantuan picnics, with starched tablecloths, a dozen impressive courses — and a staff of servants to make it all happen. Today's more casual lifestyle prefers to keep outdoor dining simple and easy, but just for a change, strike a note of formality. Pack up your picnic basket with your finest china and linens, some bottles of chilled wine and a delectable selection of foods (all prepared the day ahead, of course) and set off for the prettiest country setting you can find. Formality is not old-fashioned — it can be fun!

Unlike the Victorian picnic with its roast beef, baked hams, Melton Mowbray pies and suet puddings, our picnic features turkey or chicken breast stuffed with spinach, two interesting salads and lots of fresh fruit — definitely food of the 80s.

Analysis

Serves 8
680 calories per serving
Protein: 25%
Fat: 36%
Carbohydrate: 39%
Sodium: 700 mg
Cholesterol: 62 mg

(Photo following page 28)

Turkey Breast with Spinach Stuffing

(153 calories per serving)

All poultry is exceptionally low in saturated fat and the breast meat is the least fatty part of the bird. The spinach stuffing, reminiscent of the filling in a Greek spinach pie, helps to keep it moist. Most butchers will roll a boned turkey breast for you. Just re-open the breast, stuff and retie. Serves 8.

1 turkey breast (about 2 lbs, 1 kilo)
(or 4 chicken breasts)

Stuffing

2 teaspoons (10 mL) butter or unsaturated margarine
3 tablespoons (45 mL) finely chopped purple onion
3 tablespoons (45 mL) finely chopped leek
1 clove garlic, minced
2 cups (500 mL) fresh spinach, cleaned and chopped
3 tablespoons (45 mL) toasted pine nuts or pistachios
1 teaspoon (5 mL) lemon juice
Fat pinch of nutmeg
3 tablespoons (45 mL) feta cheese, crumbled
Pepper to taste

This dish should be made the day ahead of serving. For the stuffing, melt butter or margarine in skillet and saute onions and leeks until slightly tender. Add the rest of the ingredients and toss until spinach is slightly limp. Remove from heat and cool. Make a small slit down the centre of the poultry breasts and fill with the stuffing. Seal with skewers and tie with string to seal. Cover filling side loosely with aluminum foil and rub stuffed breasts lightly with oil. Place on rack and bake at 350 degrees F (180 degrees C). Allow about 1 hour and 30 minutes for turkey and 35 to 40 minutes for the chicken breasts, or until cooked. Cool and refrigerate.

To serve, cut off all visible fat, slice about 1/4 inch thick (6mm) and present on a dish with the cold curry sauce. Allow half a chicken breast per person, sliced on the diagonal, or 1 thin slice of turkey breast.

Curry Sauce

(38 calories per serving)

1/2 cup (125 mL) light (low calorie) mayonnaise
1/2 cup (125 mL) 2% yogurt
1 teaspoon (5 mL) curry powder, or to taste
Juice and grated zest of 1 small lime

Mix everything together and refrigerate in covered container. This keeps well so can be made several days ahead.

Salad Primavera

(147 calories per serving)

This salad is a marvellous accompaniment to barbecued fish or meats and will also complement any buffet table. It can be made a day or two ahead of serving. Vary the vegetables, depending on availability and taste.

Serves 10.

2 cups (500 mL) broccoli flowerets
1 head cauliflower, separated into flowerets
1/2 each red, yellow and green peppers, cut into julienne strips
4 medium carrots, cut into julienne strips
2 small yellow crookneck squash, sliced 1/4 inch (6 mm) thick
1/2 purple or yellow onion, thinly sliced
2 cups (500 mL) snow peas

Steam for one minute the broccoli, cauliflower, carrots and squash. String the snow peas and blanch for 30 seconds.Chill vegetables immediately afterwards in ice water and pat dry. Combine all ingredients in a large bowl and add enough of the Shallot Vinaigrette just to coat. Chill at least overnight.

Shallot Vinaigrette

4 tablespoons (60 mL) chopped shallots or green onions
2 teaspoons (10 mL) Dijon mustard
8 tablespoons (120 mL) shallot vinegar or white wine vinegar
Pepper to taste

Whisk all together and keep in refrigerator.

Oriental Noodle Salad

(150 calories per serving)

An unusual salad with a delightful flavour, this can be made the day ahead. The dressing is also great as a dip with steamed prawns or grilled chicken.

Serves 8 to 10.

1 package (300 grams) steam-fried or dry Chinese egg noodles for Chow Mein or linguine
3/4 cup (180 mL) finely chopped water chestnuts
1/2 cup (125 mL) chopped green onion
1/2 cup (125 mL) finely chopped red and yellow peppers (or 1 green pepper, finely chopped)
1 cup (250 mL) carrots, chopped and lightly steamed
3 tablespoons (45 mL) toasted sesame seeds
1/2 cup (125mL) chopped unsalted cashew nuts

Boil noodles according to directions, drain. Rinse well and toss with 1 tablespoon (15 mL) sesame oil. Mix with rest of ingredients, add dressing and toss well. Cover and refrigerate overnight.

Dressing

Serves 16.

4 tablespoons (60 mL) fresh peanut butter
*2 tablespoons (30 mL) Chinese Tamari Sauce**
2 tablespoons (30 mL) soy sauce
2 cloves garlic, crushed
4 teaspoons (20 mL) sesame oil
2 tablespoons (30 mL) rice wine vinegar or sherry
*2 tablespoons (30 mL) Red Pepper Oil***

Blend well.

* Tamari Sauce is brewed from soybeans, water and salt and contains no wheat. This gives it a different flavour from soy sauce, deep, mellow and salty-sweet.

****Red Pepper Oil**

Add 1/2 teaspoon (2 mL) red pepper flakes to 2 tablespoons (30 mL) oil, bring to boil and let sit for 5 minutes. Strain.

Sauce of the Happy Spices

(60 calories per serving)

An unusual sauce to serve with a selection of seasonal fruits. Just dip the fruits in the sauce and serve a cookie or two on the side.

Makes about 2 cups (500 mL) to serve 12 to 16.

3 tablespoons (45 mL) poppy seeds
3 tablespoons (45 mL) sunflower seeds
3 tablespoons (45 mL) sesame seeds
1 tablespoon (15 mL) mustard seeds
3/4 cup (180 mL) 2% cottage cheese, pureed
3/4 cup (180 mL) 2% yogurt, strained
1 tablespoon (15 mL) pineapple juice
1 tablespoon (15 mL) fresh lime juice
1 teaspoon (5 mL) red wine or raspberry vinegar
Grated zest of 1 lime

In a dry frying pan, lightly toast all the seeds. Cool. Blend cottage cheese and yogurt, stir in juices, vinegar and zest and fold in the seeds. This can be made a day or two ahead of serving.

Aileen's Oatmeal Hearts

(56 calories per cookie)

This healthy little cookie can be made without sugar for a great tasting savory cracker. Makes about 5 dozen.

1/2 cup (125 mL) brown sugar (optional)
1 3/4 cups (430 mL) wholewheat flour
3 cups (750 mL) rolled oats
1 teaspoon (5 mL) baking soda
Pinch salt
Pinch nutmeg
1 cup (250 mL) corn oil margarine
1 teaspoon (5 mL) vanilla
About 1/2 cup (125 mL) cold water

Mix all the dry ingredients together in a bowl. Blend in the margarine, sprinkle with vanilla and enough of the water to bind the mixture. Roll out thinly and cut into tiny heart shapes. Place on greased cookie sheet (spray with vegetable coating) and bake at 375 degrees F (190 degrees C) for 8 to 10 minutes or until golden. Cool on wire tray. These are best made at least a day or two ahead of serving. Store in sealed tins.

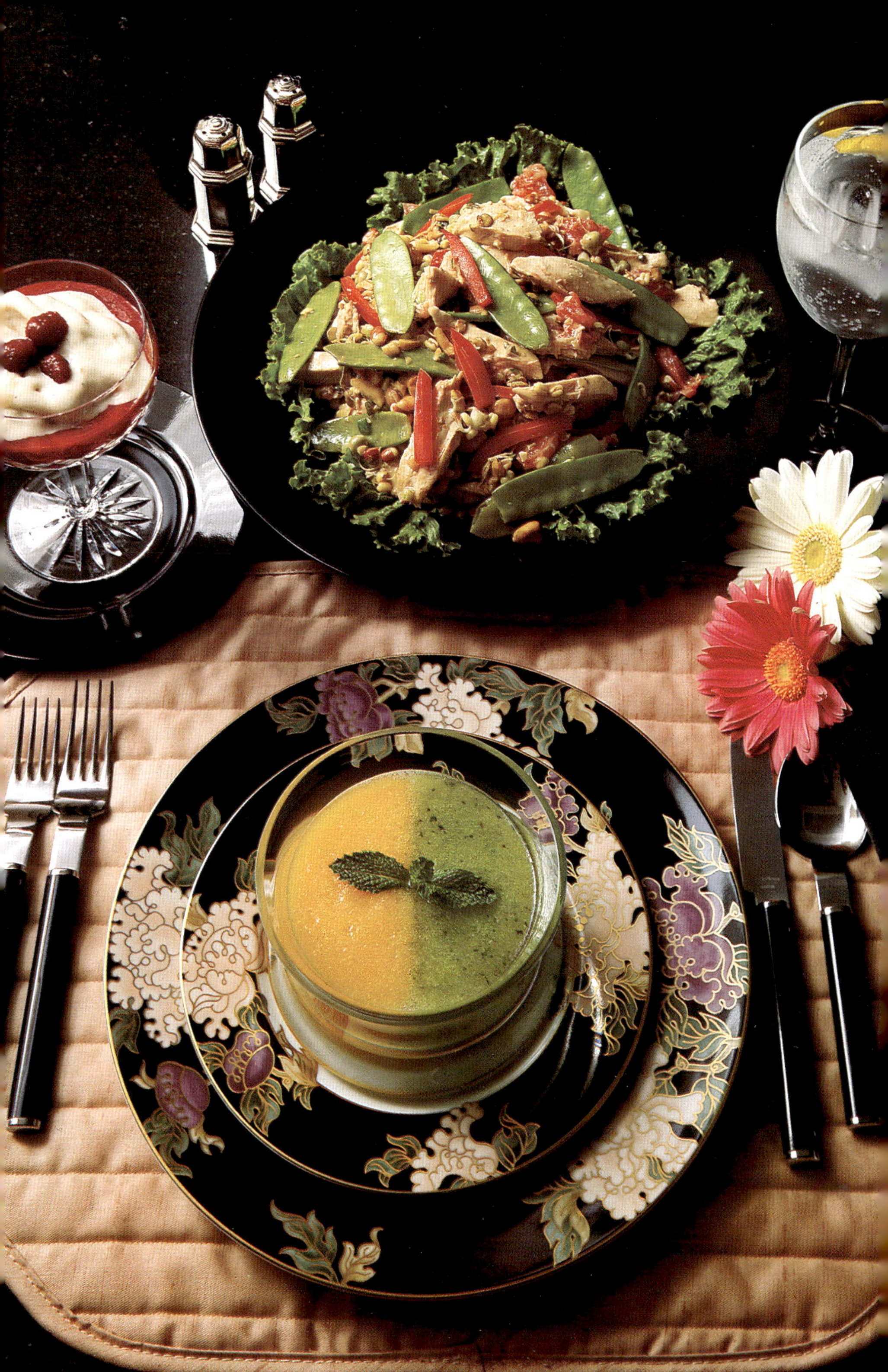

Come for Lunch, page 19. Clockwise from bottom: Chilled Melon Soup, Banana Ice with Raspberry Puree, Oriental Chicken Salad.

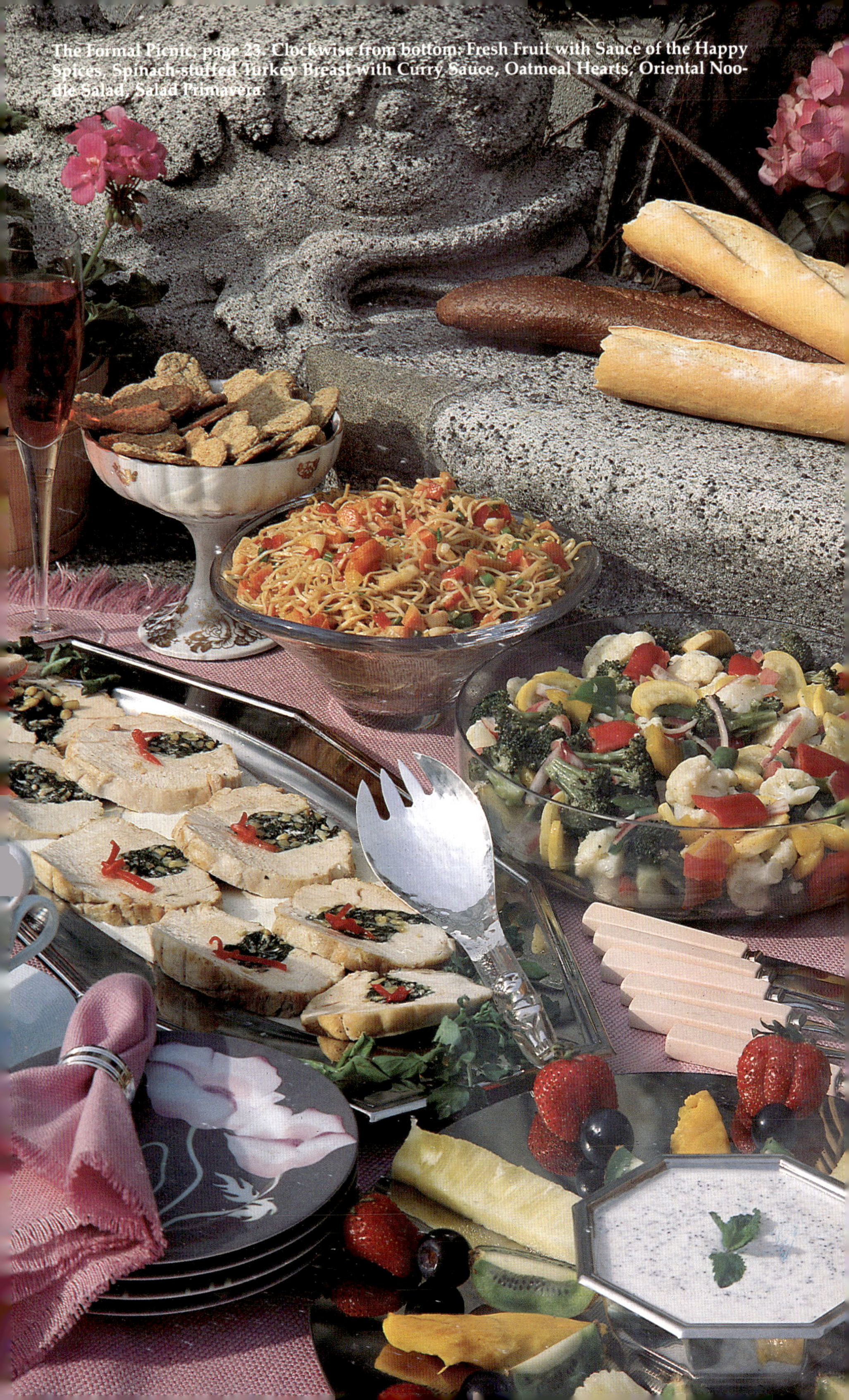

The Formal Picnic, page 23. Clockwise from bottom: Fresh Fruit with Sauce of the Happy Spices, Spinach-stuffed Turkey Breast with Curry Sauce, Oatmeal Hearts, Oriental Noodle Salad, Salad Primavera.

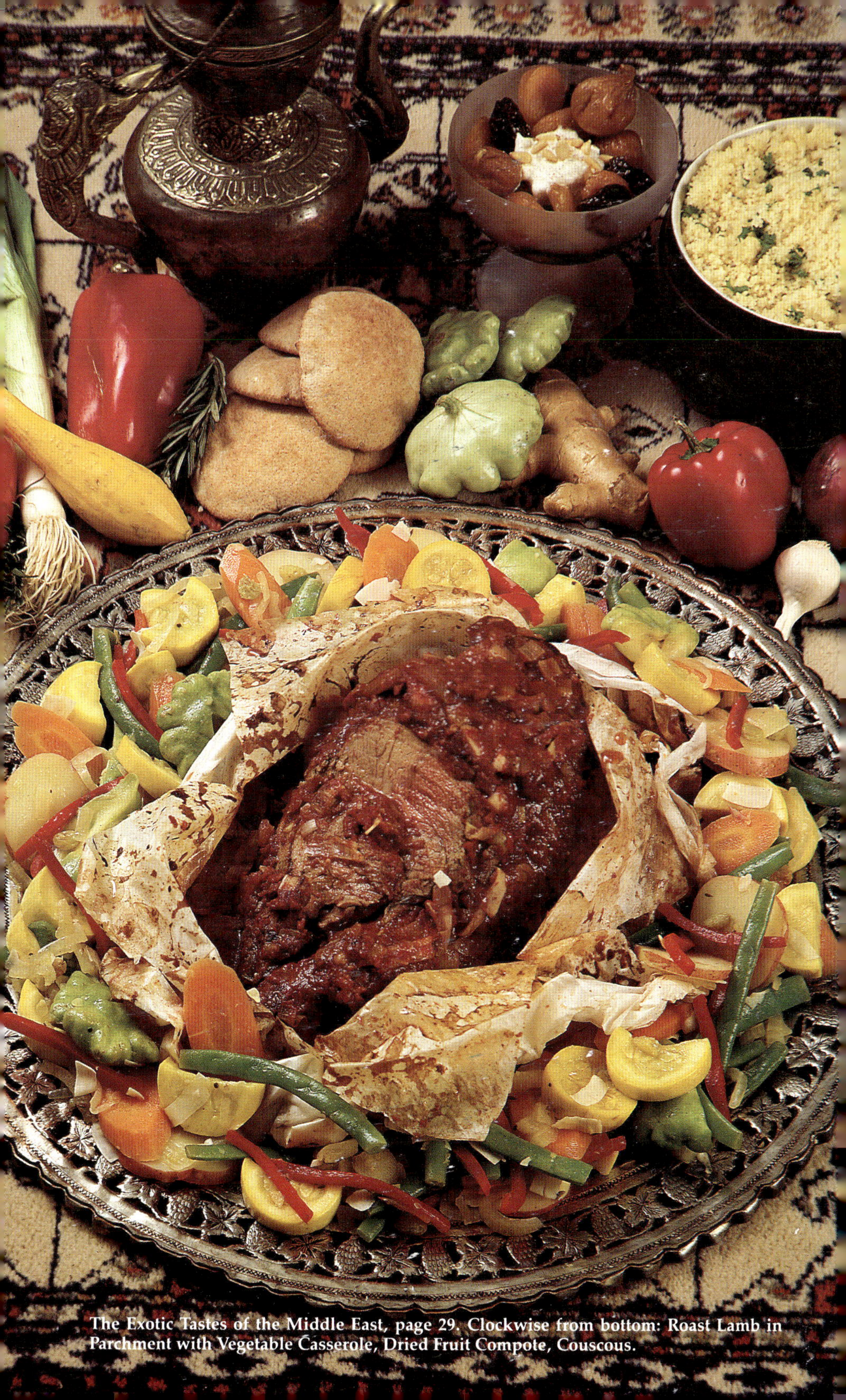

The Exotic Tastes of the Middle East, page 29. Clockwise from bottom: Roast Lamb in Parchment with Vegetable Casserole, Dried Fruit Compote, Couscous.

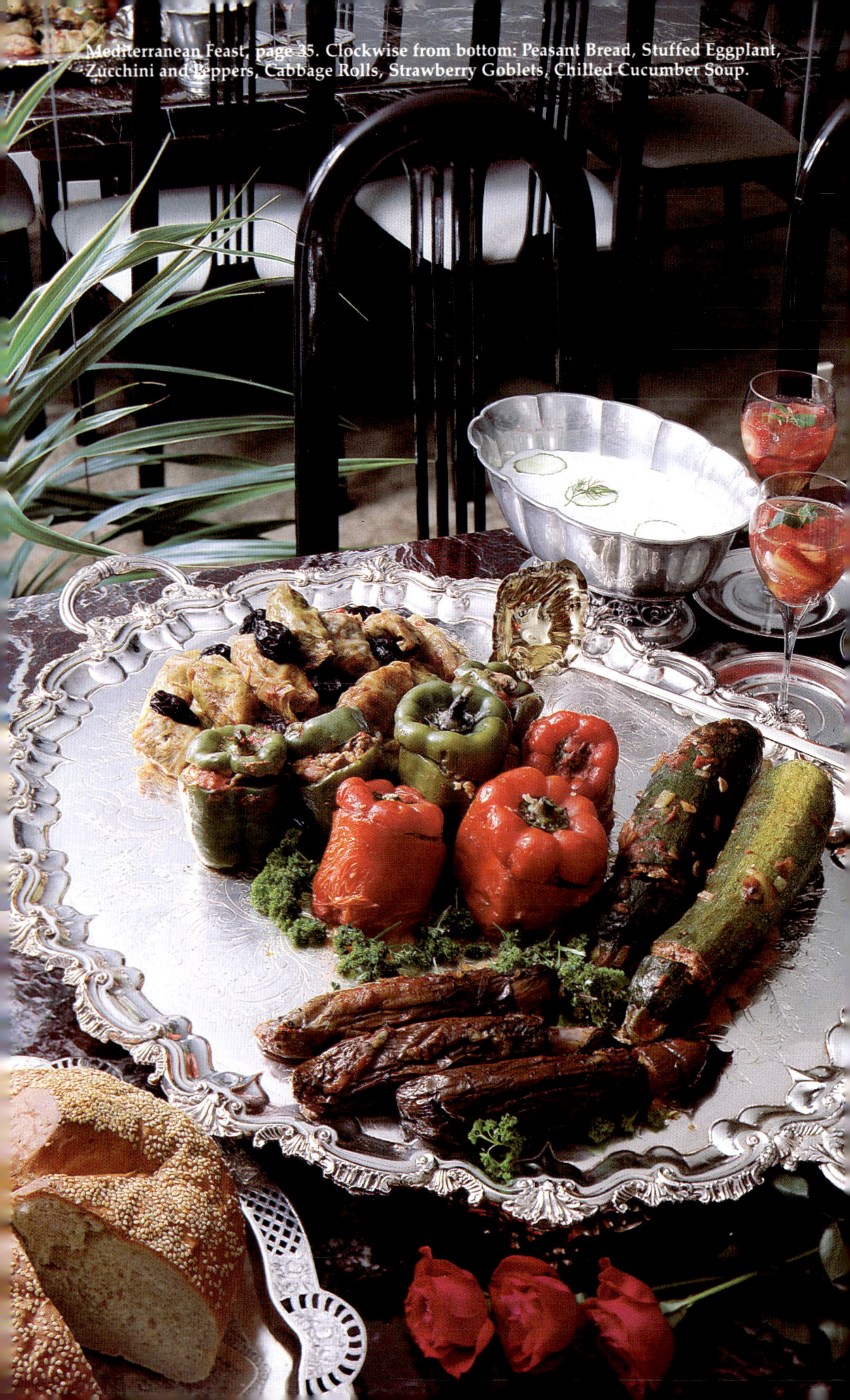

Mediterranean Feast, page 35. Clockwise from bottom: Peasant Bread, Stuffed Eggplant, Zucchini and Peppers, Cabbage Rolls, Strawberry Goblets, Chilled Cucumber Soup.

The Exotic Tastes of the Middle East

All-Season Zucchini Dill Soup

Roast Lamb in Parchment

Vegetable Casserole

Couscous

Pita Bread

Dried Fruit Compote

Spiced Coffee Mint Tea

The cuisine of the Middle East, particularly that of Lebanon, Syria and Jordan, is naturally a healthy one. Meat is not the mainstay: the focus is on whole grains, rice and beans, fresh vegetables, dried and fresh fruits and nuts along with the liberal use of such tantalizing spices as cumin, coriander and turmeric.

This menu was inspired by a memorable Moroccan Lamb and Couscous dinner served at a popular New York bistro, the Cafe Une, Deux, Trois, in the heart of the theatre district. The restaurant exuded energy, both from the staff and from the talkative theatre-crowd patrons. Its menu is creative, always dramatic in its presentation and changes daily.

All the dishes in this menu with the exception of the lamb can be prepared the day ahead of serving. The presentation should be informal.

Analysis

Serves 8
1082 calories per serving
Protein: 20%
Fat: 31%
Carbohydrate: 49%
Sodium: 458 mg
Cholesterol: 124 mg

(Photo following page 28)

All-Season Zucchini Dill Soup

(169 calories per serving)

This soup is robust and nutritious and is equally tasty served hot or chilled. Large chunks of zucchini, broccoli and leeks simmer until tender in a herbed chicken-vegetable stock, then are pureed smooth. I dress it up with a spoonful of yogurt and a pinch of chervil. The use of fresh herbs will result in a more pungent flavour. For vegetable bouillon, I use Morgan cubes from Switzerland. These should be available in health food stores or the specialty food section of your supermarket. Allow about 1/2 cup (125 mL) per serving, more if using the soup as a main meal. Serves 8 as soup course.

1 cube unsalted vegetable bouillon, dissolved in 1 quart (1 litre) water
1 quart (1 litre) home-made chicken stock (see Index)
4 medium size zucchini in large chunks
2 cups (500 mL) broccoli, stems and tops, coarsely chopped
3 leeks, white part only, cleaned and chopped
1/2 cup (125 mL) chopped white onion
1/2 cup (125 mL) chopped fresh dill (adjust to taste)
or 2 tablespoons (30 mL) dried dill
1 tablespoon (15 mL) chopped fresh chervil or parsley
or 1 teaspoon (5 mL) dried chervil
3 tablespoons (45 mL) chopped fresh basil
or 1 tablespoon (10 mL) dried basil
1 1/2 teaspoons (7 mL) fresh oregano
or 1/2 teaspoon (2 mL) dried oregano
Fresh pepper to taste
1/2 cup (125 mL) green peas, fresh or frozen

Mix together the vegetable and chicken stocks in a large Dutch oven and bring to a boil. Add all the ingredients except the peas and simmer for about 15 to 20 minutes until vegetables are tender. Add peas and simmer for a few more minutes. Cool. Strain the stock and set aside. Puree the vegetables until smooth, then mix thoroughly with the reserved stock. Adjust seasonings if necessary and refrigerate, covered.

To serve, bring soup slowly to a boil and ladle into small bowls. Add a spoonful of yogurt and a sprinkle of herbs for garnish. The soup is also excellent served cold and makes a fine meal by itself, along with a salad and a hearty whole-grain bread. For longer keeping, it freezes very well.

Roast Lamb in Parchment

(393 calories per serving)

You will really savour the aroma of this fresh leg of lamb, bathed in a spicy herb marinade, as it bakes to tender perfection in a parchment wrap. The marinade should be made the day ahead to give time for the flavours to mingle; add to the lamb just before baking. Don't forget to remove all visible fat from the meat before you start. Serves 8.

4lb (2 kilo) fresh leg of lamb
vegetable or olive oil
2 large sheets of baking parchment or foil

Marinade

2 cloves of garlic, finely chopped
1 shallot, finely chopped
1 large or 2 small leeks, white part only, cleaned and chopped
1/2 cup (125 mL) finely chopped red or white onion
3/4 cup (180 mL) dry red wine
14-oz (398 mL) can low-sodium tomato sauce or home-made tomato coulis (see Index)
1/3 cup (80 mL) sun-dried tomatoes in julienne strips or substitute 1/2 cup (125 mL) red or green peppers
4 tablespoons (60 mL) lemon juice
Chopped zest of 2 lemons
1/2 teaspoon each (2 mL) ground allspice, nutmeg, cumin and paprika
Pepper to taste

On the day ahead, combine marinade ingredients, bring to a boil and simmer for about 10 minutes. Cool. Refrigerate, covered. On the day of serving, start oven at 350 degrees F (180 degrees C). Rub both sides of the cooking parchment with oil. Make sure the parchment sheets are long enough to fully enclose the lamb when wrapped and sealed. Place one sheet of parchment in large roasting pan. Place lamb in centre and pour marinade evenly over the top. Cover with the second parchment sheet and fold and pinch the edges of both sheets together to make a tight seal. Rub parchment with more oil.

Roast for about 2 to 2 1/2 hours or until lamb is tender but not dry. It should still be pinkish in the centre. I usually find the lamb is ready after 2 hours, but ovens vary.

To serve: place parchment-wrapped lamb in the centre of a large platter and surround it with the vegetables. Slice parchment open down the middle, slice the lamb and supply plenty of couscous and pita bread to soak up the marvellous sauce.

Vegetable Casserole

(105 calories per serving)

Casseroles of mixed vegetables are popular as side or main dishes throughout the Middle East. The types of vegetables vary according to availability and the custom of the region, but it is the spices that make this dish outstanding. It is equally pleasing served hot or cold.

This dish takes a fair time to prepare but it can be made the day ahead and reheated just before serving. Don't overcook the vegetables. Crookneck and pattypan squash are particularly interesting additions.

Serves 8 to 10.

1/4 teaspoon (1 mL) each of the seeds of cumin, fennel and mustard or 1/4 teaspoon (1 mL) each of pulverized cumin, coriander and Dijon mustard
3 cups (750 mL) chicken stock
1 small onion, finely chopped
1 clove garlic, finely chopped
1 large green apple, peeled, cored and chopped
Juice and zest of 1 lemon
1/3 cup (80 mL) golden raisins
1 tablespoon (15 mL) finely minced fresh ginger root or 1 teaspoon (5 mL) dried ginger
4 or 5 small red potatoes, unpeeled, sliced 1/4-inch (6mm) thick

If using the spice seeds, first put them into a small frypan with 1 teaspoon (5 mL) oil and stir over medium heat until they start to pop. Remove seeds from pan, cool and pat dry. Add seeds and rest of ingredients except the potatoes to the chicken stock in a large skillet. Bring to a boil and simmer for about 5 minutes. Then add potatoes, sliced about 1/4 inch (6 mm) thick and

simmer for 15 to 20 minutes until they are just tender. Cool; set aside.
Steam the following vegetables separately until just tender:

1 1/2 cups (375 mL) carrots, sliced diagonally
2 crookneck squash, cut in half, if large, and sliced
4 small pattypan squash, cut into halves or quarters
1 red pepper, in julienne strips
1 1/2 cups (375 mL) fresh whole green beans

When all the vegetables are steamed to tender-crisp, add to the reserved chicken stock and potato mixture and toss lightly. Add 3 tablespoons (45 mL) of large flake coconut and refrigerate, covered, overnight. Reheat to serve.

Note: If pattypan and crookneck squash are not available, substitute zucchini.

Couscous

(108 calories per serving)

Couscous is a cereal made from coarsely ground durum wheat (semolina) which has been pre-cooked. It is a staple of North African countries where they steam it over special pots and serve with stewed meats and vegetables. Couscous can be found in Greek grocery stores as well as specialty and health food stores. I use instant couscous to save time. It works well. Serves 8.

2 cups (500 mL) instant medium couscous
2 1/2 cups (625 mL) strong chicken stock, boiling
Chopped parsley

Just before serving, combine couscous and boiling stock in a medium-sized saucepan. Cover and leave to stand for about 5 minutes. Stir to fluff up, add fresh parsley and serve as a bed for the slices of lamb, sauce and vegetables. If the couscous has to wait for some reason, reheat in a microwave oven. Try it, too, with an added pinch of saffron and a handful of raisins.

Dried Fruit Compote

(234 calories per serving)

Throughout the Middle East, dried fruits such as raisins, apricots and figs are widely used in main dishes as well as for dessert. This compote makes a perfect ending to the meal, served with spiced coffee or mint tea. Buy the freshest dried fruit available. I find the fruit in a health food store generally superior to those in supermarket packets. Serves 12 to 14.

2 cups (500 mL) canned apricot nectar
1 lb (500 grams) dried apricots
1/2 lb (250 grams) whole dried figs
1/2 lb (250 grams) pitted prunes
1/2 cup (125 mL) toasted pine nuts or almond halves
2 to 3 tablespoons (30 to 45 mL) Amaretto liqueur (optional)
Yogurt, plain or honey-sweetened.

Make this dish several days ahead for best flavour. It will keep, refrigerated, in a well-sealed container for weeks. Heat nectar to boiling in a medium-size saucepan. Add dried fruits and simmer for 15 minutes or until fruit is slightly softened. Cool. Add liqueur if desired, seal well and refrigerate.

Serve a little of each fruit and some juice in small glass bowls or wine goblets. Small portions are recommended — it's rich! Top each serving with a dollop of yogurt and sprinkle on some toasted nuts.

Spiced Coffee

In each pot of freshly brewed strong coffee, steep a few cloves, cardamom seeds and a cinnamon stick for about 5 minutes. Strain and serve.

Mint Tea

Brew a pot of herbal mint tea and float a fresh mint leaf on the top of each cup.

Mediterranean Feast

Chilled Cucumber-Yogurt Soup

Stuffed Vegetable Melange
(Cabbage Rolls, Peppers, Eggplant and Zucchini)

Hearty Peasant Bread or Wholewheat Pita Bread

Shimmering Strawberry Goblets

Haik Gharibian, a good friend who contributed to both my other cookbooks, created the main entree for this menu, a dramatic presentation of four different stuffed vegetables which reflects his Armenian heritage. For a large dinner party, serve all of them, letting guests sample each dish. For smaller affairs, cook only one or two. Each stuffed vegetable has a personality and a flavour of its own. While each takes time to make, they can be made up to a day ahead and all can cook together in the oven. The light soup and dessert can also be made ahead.

Analysis

Serves 10 to 12
785 calories per serving (combination)
Protein: 24%
Fat: 16%
Carbohydrate: 60%
Sodium: 944 mg
Cholesterol: 93 mg

(Photo following page 28)

Chilled Cucumber-Yogurt Soup

(54 calories per serving)

Kasey Wilson praised my recipe for Scalloped Oysters which she used in her Granville Island Cookbook. I happen to think her cucumber-yogurt soup is also outstanding, so here it is. Serves 6.

2 cups (500 mL) plain yogurt
1 tablespoon (15 mL) lemon juice
Zest of 1/2 lemon
1 tablespoon (15 mL) fresh mint, finely chopped
1 teaspoon (5 mL) fresh dill
or 1/2 teaspoon (2 mL) dried dillweed
2 teaspoons (10 mL) olive oil
1 garlic clove
1 teaspoon (5 mL) salt, optional
1 English cucumber, peeled and grated
1/2 cup (125 mL) chopped green onion

Place half the yogurt in blender or food processor. Add lemon juice and zest, mint, oil, garlic and salt and process for 8 seconds. Transfer to a bowl and add the rest of the yogurt and the other ingredients. Cover and chill for 4 hours. Garnish each serving with a thin slice of cucumber and a sprig of dill or a mint leaf. Substitute lime instead of lemon for a subtle different taste.

Hearty Peasant Bread

(112 calories per slice)

This crisp and chewy gluten bread is perfect for this bold dinner. It is easy to make and is best served warm. Gluten flour, which is 75% protein, can be obtained in health food stores. Makes 1 large loaf, 20 slices, to serve 8 to 10.

4 cups (1 litre) unbleached flour
1 cup (250 mL) vital gluten 80% flour
2 cups (500 mL) water
3 tablespoons (45 mL) dry yeast
2 teaspoons (10 mL) sugar
1 teaspoon (5 mL) salt
Sesame seeds

Dissolve salt, sugar and yeast in the warm water. Beat in one cup of flour, cover and leave to rise for about 30 minutes. Beat in gluten flour, then add enough of the unbleached flour to make a stiff dough. Knead until smooth and silky, about 10 minutes. Place in an oiled bowl, cover and leave to rise until double in volume, about an hour. Punch down, and knead again, adding more flour if necessary. Shape into round loaf and place on baking tray. Brush top with milk and scatter thickly with sesame seeds. Cover and leave to rise in warm place for about 20 minutes. Carefully cut deep slashes in centre of loaf to make a star, cover again and leave for an additional 20 minutes or until double in volume.

Meanwhile heat oven to 500 degrees F (260 degrees C). Place large baking tray on lower shelf and arrange one or two upturned terra-cotta flowerpot saucers on the bottom. Bake saucers for 20 minutes or until hot. Set bread on middle rack. Pour about a cup of cold water over the saucers to create steam and close oven door. Bake bread for 15 minutes, then reduce heat to 400 degrees F (200 degrees C). Wet saucers again, if necessary. Continue to cook for another 15 minutes or until loaf is nicely brown. Cool on rack and serve warm.

This bread freezes well. Thaw and reheat, well wrapped, before serving.

Cabbage Rolls

(247 calories per main meal serving, 106 as combo)

1 large white cabbage
1/2 lb (250 grams) ground veal
Pepper to taste
1/4 teaspoon (1 mL) Tabasco sauce
1 cup (250 mL) long grain rice
1/4 teaspoon (1 mL) celery seeds
4 green onions, chopped
4 tablespoons (60 mL) chopped parsley
1 cup (250 mL) tomato sauce (low sodium)
15 unpitted prunes

Separate leaves of cabbage, remove coarse ribs and steam for about 20 minutes. Mix together all the rest of the ingredients except the tomato sauce and the prunes. Place small spoonsful on the cabbage leaves and roll up jelly-roll fashion, tucking in the sides neatly. Place a layer of the rolls in a Dutch oven. Put 5 to 6 prunes and a little tomato sauce on top and cover with a second layer. Repeat until all rolls are in. Pour rest of tomato sauce on top and add 1/4 cup of water. Cover and bake at 350 degrees F (180 degrees C) for 1 hour.

Serves 6 as main entree, 14 as combo.

Stuffed Red and Green Peppers

(390 calories main entree, 111 as combo)

2 large green peppers
2 large red peppers
1/2 lb (250 mL) ground veal
Pepper to taste
4 green onions, chopped
1 cup (250 ml) yellow split peas
1/2 cup (125 mL) tomato sauce (low sodium)
2 teaspoons (10 mL) dried basil
(or 1 tablespoon (15 mL) fresh)
1 cup (250 mL) tomato sauce

Cut off tops of peppers, core and seed. Cook split peas for 15 minutes in boiling water, or soak overnight. Mix together all the ingredients except the cup (250 mL) of tomato sauce and stuff the peppers. Put peppers in a heavy pan, cover with the remaining tomato sauce plus 1/4 cup (60 mL) water, cover and bake at 350 degrees F (180 degrees C) for one hour.

Serves 4 as main entree, 14 as combo.

Stuffed Japanese Eggplant

(485 calories as main entree, 139 as combo)

Japanese eggplant are long and thin. You can find them in specialty produce sections or markets.

4 Japanese eggplants
1 7 oz (196 mL) can water chestnuts, drained and chopped
1/2 lb (250 grams) ground veal
1 cup (250 mL) bulgar wheat
4 green onions, chopped
Pepper to taste
1/2 cup (125 mL) tomato sauce (low sodium)
2 teaspoons (10 mL) dried mint
1 cup (250 mL) tomato sauce

Slice eggplants lengthwise and scoop out centres. Mix the rest of the ingredients except the cup (250 mL) of tomato sauce and stuff each eggplant half. Put halves together and seal with toothpicks.

Place in heavy dish, pour over the remaining tomato sauce and 1/4 cup (60 mL) water, cover and bake at 350 degrees F (180 degrees C) for 1 hour. Serves 4 as main entree, 14 as combo.

Stuffed Zucchini

(315 calories main meal, 135 combo)

4 to 5 large zucchini
$^1/_2$ lb (250 grams) ground veal
Pepper to taste
1 cup (250 mL) pearl barley
1 cup (250 mL) sliced mushrooms
2 teaspoons (10 mL) dried dillweed
(or 1 tablespoon (15 mL) fresh)
$1^1/_2$ cup (375 mL) tomato sauce (low sodium)
1 cup (250 mL) tomato sauce

Cut off ends of zucchini and carefully hollow them out. Mix all the ingredients except the 1 cup (250 mL) tomato sauce and stuff the zucchini, sealing the ends with aluminum foil. Place in heavy dish, cover with the remaining tomato sauce and add $^1/_4$ cup (60 mL) water. Cover and bake for 1 hour at 350 degrees F (180 degrees C).

Serves 6 as main entree, 14 as combo.

Shimmering Strawberry Goblets

(128 calories per serving)

This dessert is elegant and quick to make, a perfect summer treat, particularly when the strawberries are in season. It really does shimmer.

Serves 4 to 6.

4 cups (1 litre) white grape juice
2 tablespoons (30 mL) unflavoured gelatin
2 to $2^1/_2$ cups (500 to 625 mL) sliced fresh strawberries or raspberries

The day ahead, or on the morning of serving pour the grape juice into a large saucepan. Sprinkle gelatin on top and leave to soften for about 5 to 8 minutes. Heat the juice, stirring, over medium heat until gelatin is dissolved. Pour into a bowl and chill until the juice thickens to the consistency of unbeaten egg whites, about 50 to 60 minutes. Keep checking. Don't let it get too thick before adding the strawberries. Fold in sliced strawberries, then spoon mixture into four to six stemmed wine goblets. Chill until set.

Pasta Power

Tomato Salad
with Fresh Basil Vinaigrette

Angel Hair Pasta
with Crab, Snow Peas and Mushrooms

Cracked Wheat Rolls

Hot Apricot Souffle
with Mango Puree

Pasta is not only good, it is good for you. One cup of pasta provides 42 grams of carbohydrate, 8 grams of protein and only 1 gram of fat. It provides reasonable amounts of iron, riboflavin, niacin and thiamine — all this for only 210 calories! Add vegetables for fibre and a light sauce and you have a well-balanced food.

Pasta today comes in many different flavours, including whole wheat, tomato, spinach, beet and carrot. It also comes in numerous shapes, widths and lengths. Because of its new-found popularity, it is available fresh in many food markets.

For this menu I used angel hair pasta (super-thin spaghetti) in a light sauce topped with crab and fresh vegetables. A fresh tomato salad for starters and a delicate apricot souffle for the finale completes a full and healthy meal that can be prepared in less than half an hour.

Analysis

Serves 4
840 calories per serving
Protein: 23%
Fat: 21%
Carbohydrate: 56%
Sodium: 978 mg
Cholesterol: 47 mg

(Photo following page 60)

Tomato Salad with Fresh Basil Vinaigrette

(313 calories per serving)

This salad, which is Doug's favourite, is at its best in the summer when field-ripened tomatoes are sweet and plentiful and fresh basil is readily available.

It also goes well with grilled salmon or chicken. Serves 4.

4 ripe beefsteak tomatoes, sliced 1/4-inch (6mm) thick
4 tablespoons (60 mL) finely chopped shallots or purple onion
1/2 cup (125 mL) toasted pine nuts
A few Greek calamata olives
Fresh basil leaves
Leafy or butter lettuce

Steam shallots or onions briefly in a non-stick pan moistened with 1 teaspoon (5 mL) water or chicken stock, just to soften. Be careful they don't burn. Set aside. Arrange tomatoes and lettuce leaves on a large platter. Drizzle about 3 tablespoons (45 mL) dressing down the middle of the tomatoes, sprinkle with a little chopped fresh basil, pine nuts and cooked shallots. Sprinkle pepper to taste. Decorate with olives, whole basil leaves and red onion rings.

Dressing

(Makes 12 tablespoons, 45 calories per tablespoon)

1/2 cup (125 mL) chopped fresh basil
1 tablespoon (15 mL) red wine vinegar or shallot vinegar
1 clove garlic, crushed
Pepper
1 tablespoon (15 mL) chopped shallots or purple onion
1/4 cup (60 mL) olive or sunflower oil

Combine first five ingredients and blend well. Add oil gradually, continuing to blend until mixture is creamy. Refrigerate. This can be made the day ahead. Bring to room temperature and shake well before serving.

Pasta with Crab, Snow Peas and Mushrooms

(320 calories per serving)

Quick to make, this delectable dish is perfect for a busy day. Our son, Rand, gives this recipe his vote as the best in the book! If fresh crab is not available, shrimp works well, or try a combination of both. The sun-dried tomatoes make it extra tasty. Because the sauce has a delicate flavour, the very fine angel hair pasta works best, but fettucine would be acceptable.The sauce can be prepared a day ahead or early on the morning of serving. Prepare the vegetables in advance and saute them at the last minute. Serves 4.

Sauce

1 1/2 cups (375 mL) 2% cottage cheese
4 teaspoons (20 mL) chopped shallots or green onions
1 clove garlic, chopped
1/2 cup (125 mL) dry white wine

Combine all in a food processor or blender until smooth and creamy. It should take only a minute. Refrigerate. Just before serving, pour into a saucepan and heat very gently, stirring all the time, until it is just warm. (Be careful here, the sauce has a tendency to curdle if it is too hot.)

3/4 lb (375 grams) angel hair, fettucine or linguine pasta
4 tablespoons (60 mL) freshly grated Parmesan cheese
1 teaspoon (5 mL) oil (from the sun-dried tomatoes)
1 1/2 cups (375 mL) sliced mushrooms
3 tablespoons (45 mL) sun-dried tomatoes, chopped
(or 4 tablespoons (60 mL) fresh tomatoes, chopped)
2 cups (500 mL) fresh snow peas
Pepper to taste
1/4 lb (125 grams) fresh crab meat
(or cooked shrimp or prawns)

Cook pasta according to directions, keeping it al dente. Meanwhile, heat oil in skillet and saute mushrooms, tomatoes and snow peas until just cooked, the snow peas should be tender crisp. Pepper to taste and gently toss in the crab. Keep warm while the pasta cooks.

Drain pasta and put in serving dish. Add hot sauce and toss gently to mix. Add the crab mixture and the Parmesan cheese and toss again. Serve at once with additional Parmesan cheese. (If you have a microwave oven, quickly heat the dish through before serving.)

Hot Apricot Souffle with Mango Puree

(224 calories per serving)

Apricots are one of my favourite fruits. I love them in this light-as-a-cloud souffle cooked without egg yolks and only a little sugar. I bake it in a one-quart (1 litre) souffle dish which allows it to rise well above the rim for an elegant look and serve a little mango or other fruit puree on the side. Like all cooked souffles, it must be cooked immediately before serving but you can have the base ready, whip up the egg whites at the last minute and pop it into the oven to bake while you're eating dinner. Serves 4 to 6.

6 ounces (200 grams) dried apricots
1 cup (250 mL) unsweetened apricot nectar or orange juice
1 teaspoon (5 mL) vanilla
6 large egg whites, at room temperature
Pinch salt
1/2 teaspoon (2 mL) cream of tartar
2 tablespoons (30 mL) fine granulated sugar or fructose

Early on the day of serving, spray souffle dish with non-stick vegetable spray and make a three-inch (8 cm) collar of aluminum foil. Spray inside of collar.

In a small saucepan, cook apricots with nectar or juice for about 15 minutes or until apricots are tender. Cool and puree. Add vanilla. This will be thick and can be made the day ahead. Heat oven to 375 degrees F (190 degrees C). If the apricot base is made ahead and refrigerated, bring to room temperature. Beat egg whites until frothy, then add salt and cream of tartar and beat more until slightly stiff but still glossy. Add sugar a little at a time and beat until stiff. Fold in a little of the apricot mixture, then add the rest very gently until well blended. Pour into the souffle dish (it should come just above the rim) and bake for about 25 to 30 minutes until golden and firm to the touch. Remove foil and serve immediately with fresh pureed mangoes or other fruits.

Mango Puree

Peel, seed and chop three fresh ripe mangoes. Puree, then strain and store in refrigerator. Makes about 1/2 cup (125 mL).

In the Italian Tradition

Antipasto

Spinach Pinwheels

Italian Bread

Lemon Slush with Fresh Berries

A different twist to an old favourite, this pinwheel pasta is simply a combination of regular and spinach lasagne noodles rolled up with an iron-rich spinach filling and a fresh tomato sauce. Served in small portions, it also makes a tasty, and eye-catching, appetizer course.

This Italian dinner is light-hearted and casual, with its antipasto tray of assorted vegetables, crisp Italian bread and for dessert, a tart Italian lemon ice served with seasonal berries. If you want to expand the menu to feed a crowd, add Veal Scallopine with Lemon and Zucchini Tomato Medley (see Index).

Analysis

Serves 4
743 calories per serving
Protein: 19%
Fat: 24%
Carbohydrate: 57%
Sodium:1600 mg
Cholesterol: 42 mg

(Photo following page 60)

Antipasto

(99 calories per serving)

This easy to prepare Italian tradition is always popular. Ingredients can vary, depending on the season and what is available at your specialty stores. I try to include some of the following:

Italian green and black marinated olives
Canned baby corn
Whole artichoke hearts, not marinated. (Add a twist of lemon, some pepper, about 1 tablespoon (15 mL) olive oil and about 1 teaspoon (5 mL) vinegar and some sun-dried tomatoes or chopped purple onion.)
Canned garbanzo beans. (Mix with chopped red pepper, 1 tablespoon (15 mL) each of oil and vinegar and 1 teaspoon (5 mL) chopped parsley and green onion.)
Cherry tomatoes
Fresh shrimp

Make up your platter early in the day, cover it well and refrigerate until you are ready to serve.

Spinach Pinwheels

(450 calories per main-course serving)

This is really Lasagne-in-the-Round, but without the meat. It may not be as rich but it's certainly filling. Serve it as a first course to replace the soup or salad. It can be prepared a day ahead.

Serves 4 as main course, 8 as appetizer.

8 to 10 lasagne noodles
(4 to 5 regular, 4 to 5 spinach)
1 tablespoon (15 mL) safflower oil
3 leeks, white parts only, cleaned and chopped
3 green onions, finely chopped
1 clove garlic, pressed
1 cup mushrooms, chopped
1½ lbs (680 grams) fresh spinach, cleaned and dried
(about 6 cups, 1.5 litres)
1 small red pepper, chopped
or 2 tablespoons (30 mL) chopped pimento)
1 tablespoon (15 mL) dried basil
or 3 tablespoons (45 mL) fresh basil
1 teaspoon (5 mL) dried oregano
or 3 teaspoons (15 mL) fresh oregano
¼ cup (60 mL) wholewheat breadcrumbs
Pinch freshly grated nutmeg
3 tablespoons (45 mL) grated Parmesan cheese
½ cup (125 mL) grated low-fat Mozzarella cheese
1 egg, lightly beaten
1 cup (250 mL) low-fat ricotta cheese

Topping

1 cup (250 mL) grated low-fat Mozzarella cheese
2 tablespoons (30 mL) grated Parmesan cheese

Tomato Sauce

2 cups (500 mL) Tomato Coulis (see Index)
mixed with
1 cup (250 mL) low-sodium tomato sauce

Filling

In a large skillet, saute leeks, onions and garlic in the oil until golden; add mushrooms and saute for a few minutes until just cooked, then add red peppers. Chop spinach coarsely, add to the pan and stir until it is just limp. Add herbs, breadcrumbs, nutmeg, Parmesan and Mozzarella cheeses. Set aside to cool.

In a small bowl, combine the egg and ricotta cheese, add to the spinach mixture and refrigerate. This filling is at its best made the day before serving.

On the morning of serving, cook lasagne noodles according to package directions to the al dente stage. Strain, rinse in cold water and pat dry then set them out on a work surface. Divide the spinach filling equally among them, spreading it over the entire surface of each noodle. (For each roll you will need 2 1/2 to 3 tablespoons (35 to 45 mL) of filling.) Roll each noodle up like a jelly roll.

Spread a thin layer of tomato sauce over the bottom of a large lasagne dish and place the rolls in a single layer on top. Cover each roll with additional sauce and sprinkle with some of the topping cheeses. Cover and refrigerate until ready to serve. Bake uncovered at 350 degrees F (180 degrees C) for 35 to 45 minutes or until bubbly. This dish can be made up the day ahead and heated, without the topping cheeses, for about 20 minutes, then refrigerated. The next day, add the cheeses and reheat as above.

To serve, simply spoon the rolls onto the plates from the serving dish. For a more elegant presentation, cut each roll in half and stand them on a bed of tomato sauce. Reheat and serve either on individual dishes or a serving platter with a green garnish.

Lemon Slush with Fresh Berries

(98 calories per serving)

Street vendors selling ices are as much a part of the Italian street scene as the honking Fiats. Italian ice is a far cry from North American ice-cream — it's tart and refreshing and so popular that Italian ice-cream parlours are springing up in cities around the world. Italian ice is so easy to make and you don't need an ice-cream maker. It contains no fat so it is better for you than ice cream.

In late summer, serve it with fresh blackberries for a unique flavour combination; blueberries, raspberries and strawberries are also good. This should be made the night before, or early on the morning of serving.

Serves 8.

3 cups (750 mL) water
3/4 cup (180 mL) fructose
Juice and grated zest of 4 lemons

In a medium-sized saucepan mix the water and fructose and bring to a rolling boil. Add lemon juice and zest and cool. Pour into a shallow dish and freeze. Do not stir. It's ready when a spoon still goes easily into the middle. Stir just before serving.

If you make it the night before it will freeze hard. Take it out about ten minutes before serving and mash it well. It should be slightly mushy, to melt in your mouth. Serve it in small quantities: it is very tart. For a special occasion, serve the ice in wine goblets and pour over a little well-chilled medium-dry sparkling white wine and a slice of lemon.

Light and Elegant

Stuffed Pea Pods with Scallops and Shrimps

Veal Scallopine with Lemon

Zucchini-Tomato Medley

Risotto

Assorted Breads

Tropical Mousse

Today's style of home entertaining is much less formal than it used to be. Many kitchens are now deliberately opened to the dining area so that the cook can create special dishes in front of the guests — or the guests can lend a hand. This menu lends itself well to this type of casual entertaining. Many of the dishes can be prepared ahead of time, including the pea pods which double as appetizer and salad course, the vegetable and the dessert. That leaves only the veal dish and the risotto to complete when your guests arrive. Let them take turns stirring the risotto while you work on the veal. Pass the appetizer, pour the wine — and let the party begin.

Analysis

Serves 6
669 calories per serving
Protein: 25%
Fat: 36%
Carbohydrate: 39%
Sodium: 492 mg
Cholesterol: 104 mg

(Photo following page 60)

Stuffed Pea Pods with Scallops and Shrimps

(48 calories per serving)

These pods are crunchy and tasty, with a creamy filling. Served cold on a bed of alfalfa sprouts, they serve for both appetizer and salad. Serves 6.

About 12 baby shrimp, halved
3 large scallops, cut into about 24 small pieces
20 to 24 sugar pea pods
Extra shrimp and scallops for garnish
Alfalfa sprouts

Filling

1/3 cup (80 mL) goat cheese
1 tablespoon (15 mL) ricotta cheese
1/4 teaspoon (1 mL) each dried basil, oregano and marjoram or 3/4 teaspoon (3 mL) fresh herbs, chopped
1 tablespoon (15 mL) finely chopped parsley
Pepper to taste
1/8 teaspoon (.5 mL) Dijon mustard
1/2 teaspoon (2 mL) white wine vinegar
1/2 teaspoon (2 mL) fresh lime or lemon juice

On the day ahead, combine all filling ingredients, mixing until creamy. Refrigerate overnight. Poach scallops in a little water and lemon juice, just until opaque. Cut into small pieces, refrigerate.

On the morning of serving, cut tips off peas and string them, if necessary. Blanch them in boiling water for only a few seconds, then strain and transfer to a bowl of ice water. When chilled, strain and pat dry, slice open along the top, remove the tiny peas and dry the insides. Stuff pea pods, dividing the filling evenly between them. Place shrimp half on centre of filling, with pieces of scallop on either side. Arrange stuffed pods on a bed of alfalfa sprouts and decorate with thin strips of pimento or red peppers and any leftover shrimps or scallops. Cover with plastic wrap and refrigerate until serving time.

Veal Scallopine with Lemon

(212 calories per serving)

This classic veal dish takes only minutes to prepare and can be done the day ahead or early on the morning of serving. But I like to get my guests involved. All the preparations are done in advance then I start the veal cooking while the risotto is being stirred. As you complete each batch of veal, keep it warm in the oven. The best veal to use for this dish is cut from the top sirloin. Ask your butcher to cut it thinly and pound it flat to make the ''escalopes''. The lemon glaze is tart and just lightly coats the veal. Serves 6.

18 paper-thin escalopes of veal, about 12 oz, 375 g
(allowing three per person)
1/3 to 1/2 cup (80 to 125 mL) wholewheat flour
Pepper to taste
1 tablespoon (15 mL) safflower oil
1 tablespoon (15 mL) butter
2 tablespoons (30 mL) lemon juice
1/2 cup (125 mL) white wine
Chopped parsley
Lemon wedges

Roll the veal in the flour, shaking off excess. Heat oil and butter in a nonstick frypan and saute veal, a few slices at a time, for about one minute on each side or until just golden and cooked. Don't overcook them as they soon toughen. Set aside in the oven to keep warm while you saute the rest of the veal. When all is done, add lemon juice and wine to the pan and deglaze , reducing the glaze slightly. Pour glaze over the veal, sprinkle with parsley and pepper and serve garnished with lemon wedges. If you choose to make it ahead, reheat, covered, in microwave or regular oven just until warm.

Risotto with Mushrooms and Cheese

Another Italian classic, this rice is distinguished by its creamy yet slightly crunchy texture. This comes from the type of rice, a stubby grain known as Arborio, found in Italian specialty stores and most grocery chains. To fit with today's lighter cuisine, I have reduced the amount of butter traditionally called for in this recipe.

It's a basic dish: you can change its flavour by adding saffron, seafood such as shrimps, mussels or smoked salmon, or peas and mushrooms. (Add about 3/4 cup (180 mL) of seafood when you add the last cup (150 mL) of stock, along with about 1/4 teaspoon (1 mL) of saffron and about 1/2 (125 mL) of peas. This then becomes a meal in itself. Serves 6.

3 to 3 1/4 cups (750 to 800 mL) mild chicken stock
1 cup (250 mL) Arborio rice
1 clove garlic
3 tablespoons (45 mL) chopped shallots or green onions
1 tablespoon (15 mL) butter
3 tablespoons (45 mL) freshly grated Parmesan cheese
1 cup (250 mL) sliced shiitake or regular button mushrooms, thinly sliced

In a small saucepan, heat the stock and keep it warm. Just before serving, heat the butter in a heavy saucepan and add the shallots or green onions and saute them until golden. Add rice and stir over medium heat until rice turns opaque, stirring constantly. Then start adding the warm stock, about 3/4 cup (180 mL) at a time, stirring frequently. Don't add more stock until the previous addition is almost absorbed by the rice, but don't let it stick on the pan bottom. Keep adding stock until it is all absorbed and the rice is tender, about 25 to 30 minutes. The rice should be tender and slightly creamy, though firm to the bite.

Add the cheese, toss. Add pepper to taste. In a non-stick skillet, add about ½ teaspoon (2 mL) butter and saute the mushrooms until tender. Cover skillet with a lid and let them steam for a bit. This will take only a few minutes, regardless of what variety of mushrooms you are using. Sprinkle with pepper and toss into the cooked rice. Serve immediately.

Any leftover risotto can be reheated as a pancake the next day. Moisten a non-stick frypan with a little oil, add the risotto, patting down well as if you were making hash brown potatoes. Cook over medium heat for about 6 to 8 minutes or until rice is hot and slightly golden. Serve in wedges, sprinkled with a little extra Parmesan cheese.

Zucchini Tomato Medley

(41 calories per serving)

This colourful vegetable dish is so simple to make but it goes well with the veal and risotto (and also with grilled chicken and seafood). For something simpler, serve fresh asparagus instead. Serves 6 to 8.

3 firm, medium-size tomatoes, sliced 1/4 inch (6mm) thick
1/2 purple onion, cut into rings
3 zucchini, sliced 1/8 inch (3 mm) thick
pepper
generous sprinkling of basil and oregano
About 1/2 tablespoon (7 mL) oil
1 tablespoon (15 mL) grated Parmesan cheese

Spray shallow casserole dish with oil and lay alternate slices of tomato, onion and zucchini to cover. Brush with a little oil and sprinkle with a little pepper, herbs and cheese. Refrigerate, covered, until ready to bake. Bake uncovered at 350 degrees F (180 degrees C) for about 30 minutes or until hot. This can also be served cold as a salad.

Tropical Mousse

(129 calories per serving)

Almost a pina colada, this dessert version of the popular drink is dynamite. Serve with slices of kiwi and pineapple. This can be made the day ahead. Serves 6.

1/4 cup (60 mL) unsweetened pineapple juice
1 tablespoon (15 mL) unflavoured gelatin
1 small can frozen limeade, thawed but not diluted
2 tablespoons (30 mL) canned cream of coconut or 2 tablespoons (30 mL) lime juice
1 tablespoon (15 mL) white or dark rum
1 cup (250 mL) low-fat yogurt
3 egg whites
Pinch of cream of tartar
1/2 cup (125 mL) unsalted pistachio nuts

Peel and chop pistachio nuts and roast in medium oven for about 5 minutes. Spray a two-cup (500 mL) mould with oil. Combine pineapple juice and gelatin in a small saucepan, stir until smooth, then let sit until it starts to firm. Turn heat to low and stir well until it melts. Add limeade, cream of coconut and rum and chill until it is thick, about the consistency of egg whites, about 30 minutes. Check often: it should not be allowed to get too stiff. Fold in yogurt, creaming well. Whip egg whites until foamy, add cream of tartar and whip until really stiff. Fold a little of the gelatin mixture into the egg whites, then fold in the rest. Do not overmix: there should still be a few streaks of white remaining. Pour into prepared mould and leave to set overnight.

To serve: unmould onto a platter, sprinkle with the roasted pistachio nuts and serve with slices of kiwi and pineapple.

Dinner on the Run

Walnut Blue Cheese Salad

Papillote of Seafood
with Tomatoes and Zucchini

Sourdough Bread

Steamed Vegetables

Chocolate Souffle with Mocha Sabayon

This menu takes only as much time to prepare as a Twenty Minute Workout. The presentation en papillote is dramatic — everyone enjoys cutting open the puffy surprise package — yet it is quick and simple. The salad starter is nippy and crunchy and the steamed vegetables can be prepared in advance and reheated on medium heat on top of the stove or in the microwave oven. Pop the light, low-calorie souffle into the oven just before you sit down to eat.

Analysis

Serves 6
497 calories per serving
Protein: 25%
Fat: 32%
Carbohydrate: 43%
Sodium: 433 mg
Cholesterol: 161 mg

(Photo following page 60)

Walnut Blue Cheese Salad

(200 calories per serving)

For this, it's important to use fresh walnuts and a good quality French blue cheese that crumbles easily. The blue cheese flavour is very mild so that even those who shy away from pungent cheeses will enjoy it. Use Spartan apples for colour, or Granny Smiths. Serves 6.

2 to 3 heads romaine lettuce
1/2 cup (125 mL) fresh walnuts, halved or in large pieces
3 tablespoons (45 mL) blue cheese, crumbled
2 medium apples, cored and cubed

Dressing

1/4 cup (60 mL) vegetable oil
3 tablespoons (45 mL) sherry wine vinegar
Pepper to taste

Clean and dry lettuce, break into bite-sized pieces and use it to line a large salad bowl. Toss together the walnuts, cheese and apples with a bit of the dressing and spoon into the centre of the bowl. Drizzle over just enough dressing to coat the greens and sprinkle with pepper. Serve with sourdough bread or Baguette Crisps (see Index).

Papillote of Seafood with Tomatoes and Zucchini

(76 calories per serving)

The seafood can be varied according to availability. Cooking parchment, available from kitchen boutiques, can be substituted for the aluminum foil and is actually more traditional. Be careful not to overcook the fish.

Serves 6.

$1^1/_4$ cups (300 mL) Tomato Coulis (see Index)
12 mussels or clams, cleaned
6 small pieces of sole, red snapper, cod or salmon
12 prawns, cleaned but unpeeled
16 mushrooms, sliced
2 zucchini, thinly sliced into 24 strips
1 purple or white onion, thinly sliced
1 lemon, sliced thinly and halved
6 fresh spigs of tarragon, basil, thyme or oregano

A few hours ahead of baking, fold into halves 6 pieces of cooking parchment or heavy aluminum foil, each about 15 by 20 inches (40 by 50 cms). Cut each into a Valentine heart shape (each heart should have a fold in the middle). Open hearts out and spray lightly with vegetable coating. Place 3 tablespoons (45 mL) of tomato base in the centre of each half, place fish on top and cover with 4 strips of zucchini. Arrange the rest of the ingredients around the fish, place fresh herb sprig in the centre and sprinkle with pepper. Fold over the other halves of the hearts and seal the open edges with a double fold.

Bake at 450 degrees F (225 degrees C) for 8 to 10 minutes or until the mussels or clams open. (Throw away any that don't open.) Put each papillote in a large soup or pasta bowl, slit open down the centre and spread open. Add the steamed vegetables to the bowl so they will absorb the tasty juices.

Note: If you are not using Tomato Coulis as your base, peel, seed and chop 3 to 4 tomatoes to make $1^1/_4$ cups (300 mL) and add 1 teaspoon (5 mL) dry white wine, $^1/_2$ teaspoon (2 mL) dried or $1^1/_2$ teaspoon (7 mL) each of fresh basil and oregano.

Chocolate Souffle

(159 calories per serving)

This recipe comes from Glenys Morgan of Tools and Techniques, a kitchen boutique in West Vancouver where I teach. It's lighter in calories than most souffles but you still get the satisfying taste of chocolate. The souffle must be made at the last moment but the sabayon can be prepared earlier in the day.

Serves 6.

8 or 9 large egg whites
9 tablespoons (135 mL) unsweetened cocoa, preferably Dutch
9 tablespoons (135 mL) fructose or berry sugar
1 1/2 teaspoons (7 mL) cinnamon
1 1/2 teaspoons (7 mL) vanilla
1 1/2 teaspoons (7 mL) rum
Butter for the ramekins
Cocoa for dusting

Butter six individual ramekins and lightly dust with cocoa. Place inside a larger dish and pour in enough hot water to come 2/3 up the sides of the ramekins. Preheat oven to 350 degrees F (180 degrees C).

Beat egg whites until stiff peaks form. Mix together thoroughly the sugar and the cocoa and gently fold into the whites using a rubber spatula. Fold in vanilla and rum and fill each ramekin 3/4 full. Bake 30 minutes and serve immediately with a dusting of icing sugar or Mocha Sabayon. Fresh strawberries or raspberries would go beautifully as well.

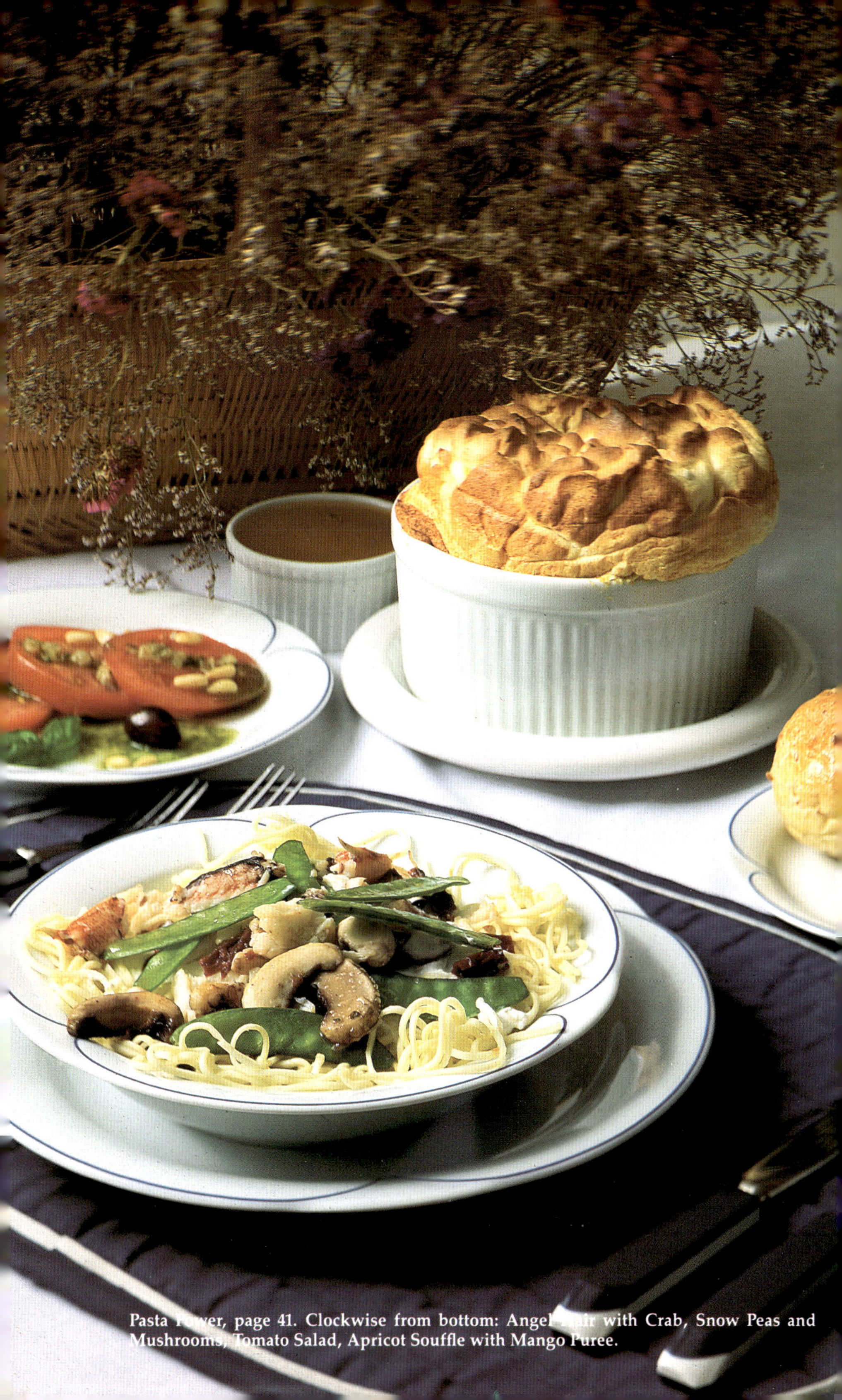

Pasta Power, page 41. Clockwise from bottom: Angel Hair with Crab, Snow Peas and Mushrooms, Tomato Salad, Apricot Souffle with Mango Puree.

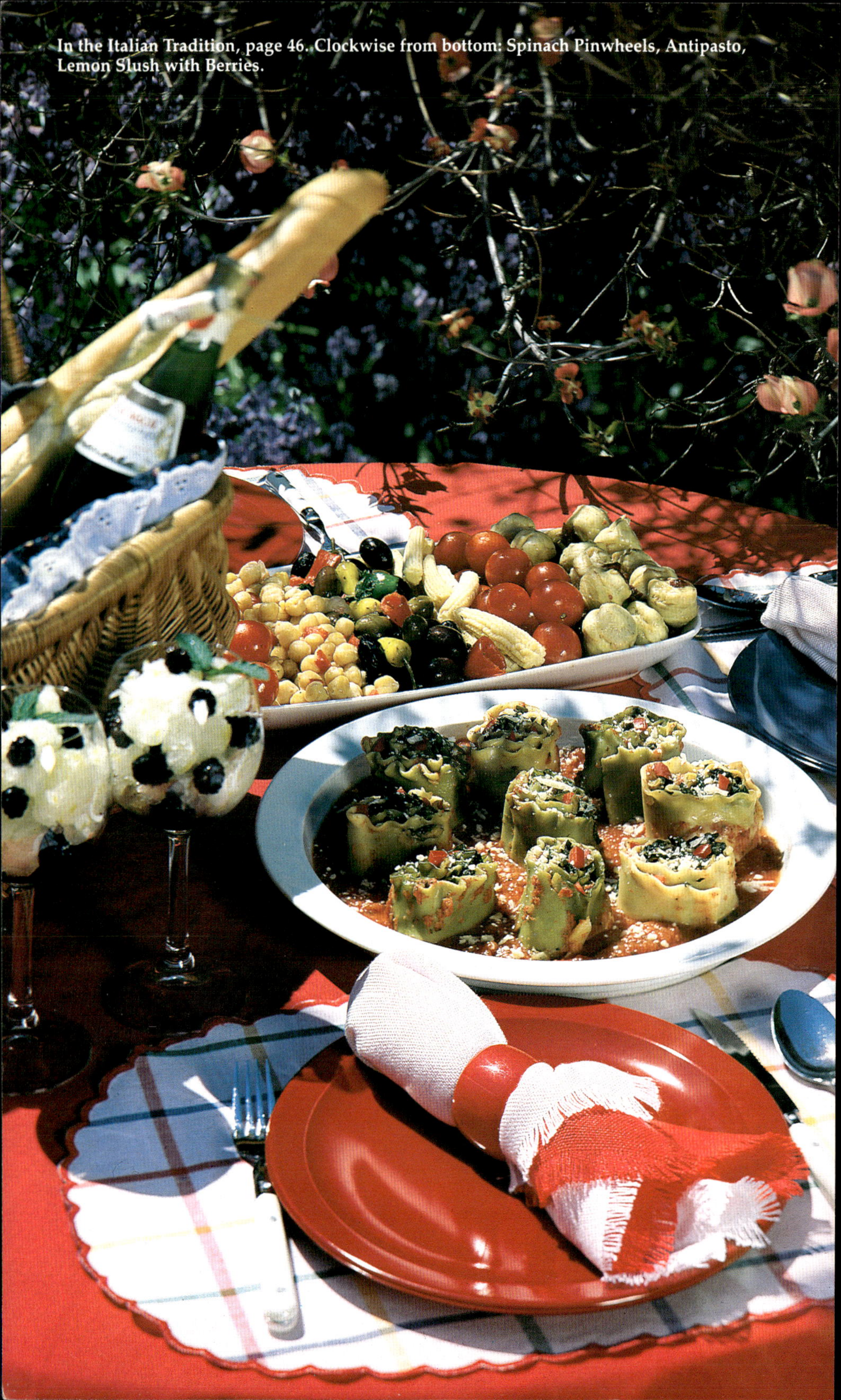

In the Italian Tradition, page 46. Clockwise from bottom: Spinach Pinwheels, Antipasto, Lemon Slush with Berries.

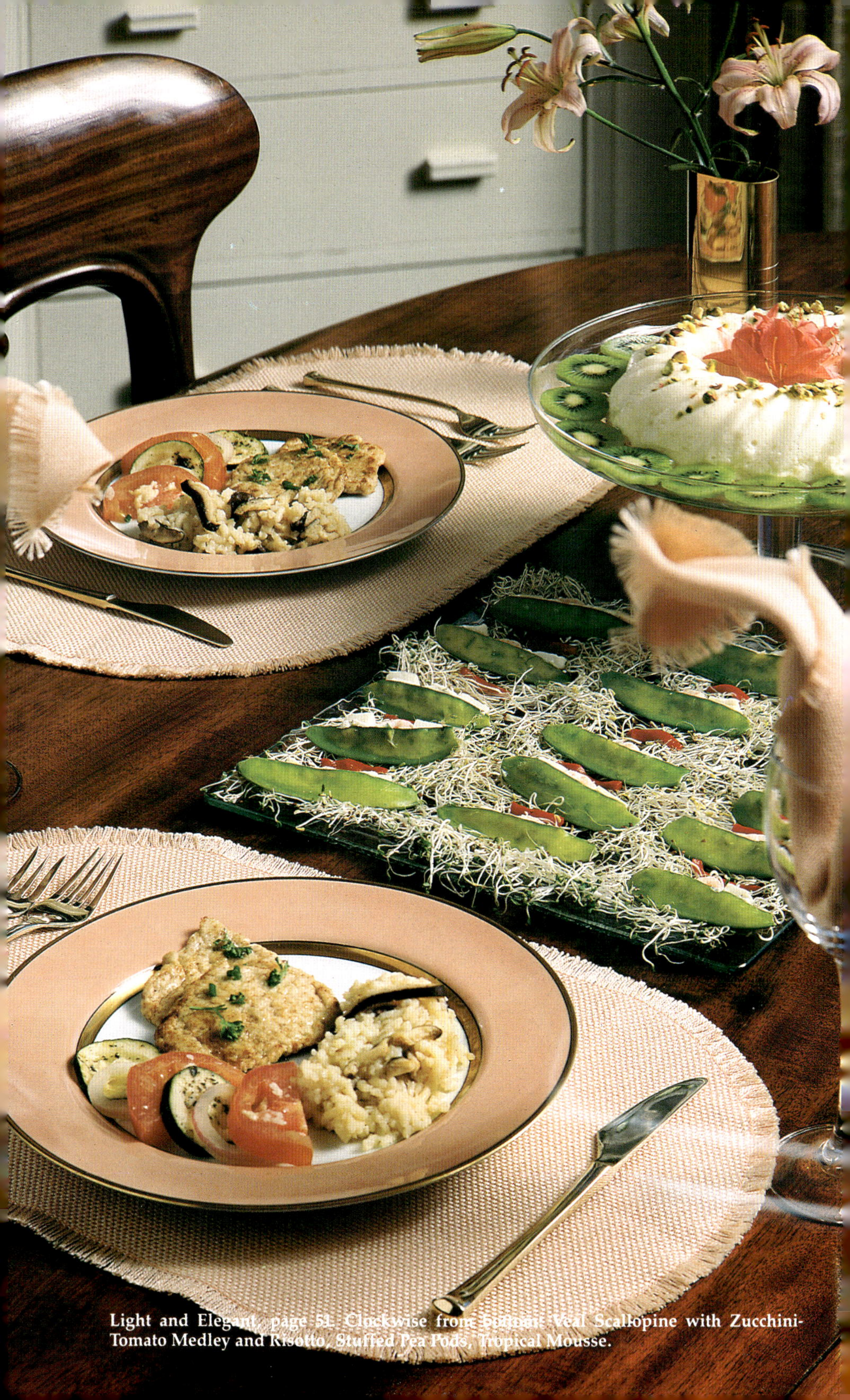

Light and Elegant, page 51. Clockwise from bottom: Veal Scallopine with Zucchini-Tomato Medley and Risotto, Stuffed Pea Pods, Tropical Mousse.

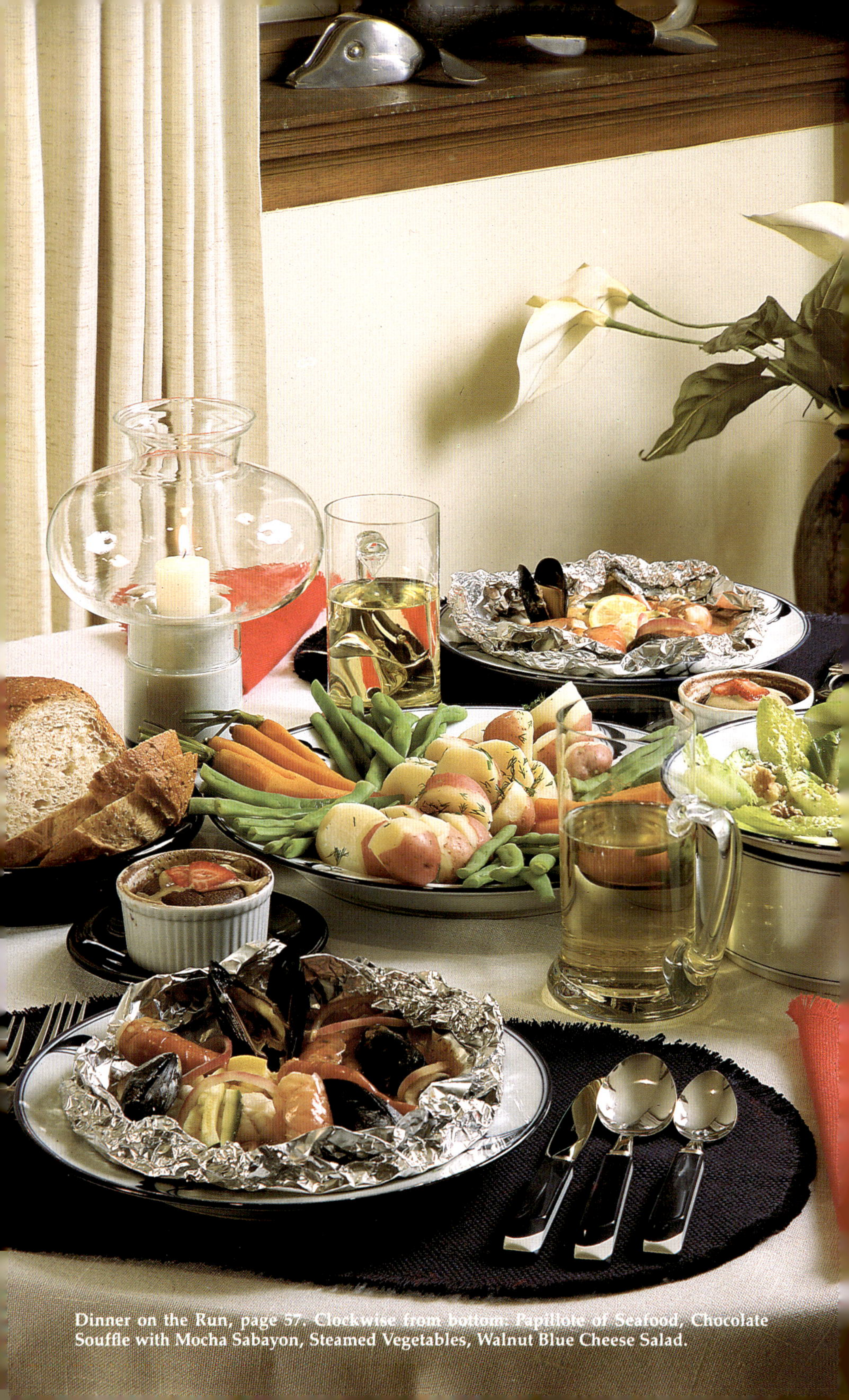

Dinner on the Run, page 57. Clockwise from bottom: Papillote of Seafood, Chocolate Souffle with Mocha Sabayon, Steamed Vegetables, Walnut Blue Cheese Salad.

Mocha Sabayon

(26 calories per tablespoon)

This recipe with its six egg yolks is rich and high in cholesterol, but you only need a spoonful or two per person.

Makes 2 cups (500 mL), enough for 12 to 16 people.

6 egg yolks
4 tablespoons (60 mL) sugar
2/3 cup (160 mL) strong coffee, preferably espresso (or mix 2 tablespoons (30 mL) instant espresso with 2/3 cup (160 mL) hot water
6 tablespoons (90 mL) cognac or brandy

In a double boiler combine egg yolks and sugar and whisk until the mixture doubles in volume. It should be creamy and thick enough to coat a spoon. Add cognac, pour into a small pitcher and serve with the hot soufles. The sabayon can be made ahead of time, but for best results, make it at the last minute. Serve warm or at room temperature.

The Contented Sole

Gazpacho

Stuffed Sole with Shrimp and Citrus Fruits

Pommes Parisienne

Fresh Asparagus

Puree of Carrots and Yams

Wholewheat or Cracked Wheat Rolls

Chocolight Cake with Strawberries

Fish has many positive qualities. It's high in calcium and protein, low in fat. It's quick to prepare and the simpler methods of preparation will result in a more succulent dish. This combination of sole stuffed with shrimp, grapefruit and oranges with just a waft of ginger, is complemented by an intense shallot-citrus sauce.

The menu gets off to a nippy start with a healthy gazpacho. Simple vegetables accompany the sole (the carrot and yam puree is optional) and the dessert is a delicate chocolate angel cake served with fresh strawberries.

Analysis

Serves 4
628 calories per serving
Protein: 24%
Fat: 18%
Carbohydrate: 58%
Sodium: 617 mg
Cholesterol: 100 mg

(Photo following page 92)

Gazpacho

(61 calories per serving)

I keep this soup on hand to served chilled during the summer. It seems to get better the longer it sits in the refrigerator. This recipe is similar to the Gazpacho in ''Chef on the Run'', but with a few extra ingredients for a new taste. Serves 8 to 10.

4 large ripe tomatoes, cored
1 14-oz (398 mL) can tomatoes, drained
1/2 medium purple or white onion
1 14-oz (398 mL) can artichoke hearts, not marinated, drained
1 English cucumber, unpeeled
or 1 regular cucumber, peeled
3 stalks celery
1 small red or green pepper, seeded, ribbed and chopped
3 tablespoons (45 mL) sun-dried tomatoes, thinly sliced
6 sprigs parsley
1 clove garlic, crushed
1 10-oz (284 mL) can V-8 Juice
2 cups (500 mL) low sodium tomato juice
1/2 tablespoon (7 mL) lemon juice
1/4 to 1/2 cup (60 to 125 mL) chili sauce, to taste
1 tablespoon (15 mL) balsamic or red wine vinegar
1/4 teaspoon (1 mL) Worcestershire Sauce
1/2 teaspoon (2 mL) dried basil
or 1 1/2 teaspoons (7 mL) fresh basil
1/4 teaspoon (1 mL) dried oregano
or 1 teaspoon (5 mL) fresh oregano
1/2 teaspoon (2 mL) Hungarian sweet paprika

At least three days before serving, cut tomatoes, onions, artichokes, cucumber, celery, and pepper into chunks and put them through a food processor or chop in a blender with the sun-dried tomatoes, parsley, garlic, V-8 and tomato juices. Add rest of ingredients and blend. Do not over-process for the mixture should be chunky. Cover and refrigerate. It will keep for up to a week. If you prefer a thinner soup, add more tomato juice and experiment with herbs and seasonings until the taste is to your liking.

Stuffed Sole with Citrus

(212 calories per serving)

The sauce can be made the day ahead and the sole prepared on the morning of serving. It takes only minutes to bake. Buy fresh sole if available and ask for wide, even fillets to hold the stuffing, allowing one fillet per person. (If the fillets are small, serve two.) Serves 4.

4 small fresh sole fillets
1/3 cup (80 mL) fresh baby shrimp
1/4 cup (60 mL) fresh orange sections
1/4 cup (60 mL) fresh grapefruit sections

Sauce

2 teaspoons (10 mL) unsalted butter
3 tablespoons (45 mL) finely chopped shallots or green onions
2 tablespoons (30 mL) dry white wine
1/2 teaspoon (2 mL) minced fresh ginger
1 1/4 cups (300 mL) mixed orange and grapefruit juice

To make the sauce, melt butter in a small skillet, add shallots or onions and ginger and saute gently until golden. Add wine, simmer for a few seconds, add 1/2 cup (125 mL) of the juice and turn heat to high. Cook until sauce is reduced to about half. Add the rest of the juice and reduce again until about 2/3 cup (160 mL) of sauce remains. Stir frequently. Cool, then refrigerate.

Early on the day of serving, spray a shallow oven-proof dish with vegetable oil. Mix shrimps with orange and grapefruit sections. Lay out the fillets, white fleshy side down (this will prevent the rolls from breaking apart when cooking), and divide the shrimp mixture evenly between them, spreading it on the widest ends of the fillets. Roll up, jelly roll fashion and place in prepared dish. Squeeze a little orange juice over all and cover with a lightly buttered piece of parchment or aluminum foil. Refrigerate until ready to bake.

Bake at 450 degrees F (230 degrees C) for about 10 minutes or until fish is just opaque. Meanwhile, heat sauce. Serve each fillet with a glaze of hot sauce on top.

Pommes Parisienne

(117 calories per serving)

These classic French-style potatoes are cooked with minimum fat and can be partially prepared the day ahead. Serves 4.

4 medium potatoes, peeled and soaked in ice water
1 teaspoon (5 mL) butter
1/2 teaspoon (2 mL) safflower oil
3 tablespoons (45 mL) chopped parsley
Pepper

On the day ahead shape out enough potato balls with a melon cutter to allow five per person. Keep in bowl of ice water to prevent discoloration. When balls are made, drop them into a pot of boiling water and simmer for about two minutes. Drain, cool and store, covered, in the refrigerator.

To serve, heat butter and oil in a non-stick skillet. Add potato balls and toss back and forth for about 5 minutes until they are golden all over and completely cooked. Add chopped parsley and pepper just before serving. These are also great served with fresh dill.

Puree of Carrots and Yams

(107 calories per serving)

Carrots are high in Vitamin C and their fibre content helps to lower cholesterol levels. Yams and sweet potatoes are high in Vitamin A and contain more calcium, iron, potassium and niacin than white potatoes. (The average yam or sweet potato provides about 135 calories.)

This puree is an unusual marriage of these two popular vegetables. Egg whites gives it the texture of a souffle but it is equally successful without them. For added flavour and texture, add a ripe banana. It can be assembled the day ahead but fold in the egg whites and the banana just before baking.

Serves 6 to 8.

3 large yams or sweet potatoes
6 large carrots
2 tablespoons (30 mL) undiluted orange juice concentrate
2 tablespoons (30 mL) finely chopped shallots or green onions
1/2 teaspoon (2 mL) cinnamon
1/2 teaspoon (2 mL) mace
1/2 teaspoon (2 mL) powdered ginger
1 teaspoon (5 mL) orange zest
1 ripe banana, mashed (optional)
3 egg whites, stiffly beaten (optional)
1/4 cup (60 mL) toasted chopped pine nuts

A day ahead, boil the yams in their jackets for 25 minutes or until tender. Cool, peel and chop into chunks. Peel, chop and steam carrots until tender. Put yams, carrots and all the ingredients except egg whites and nuts into a food processor or blender and cream well. Refrigerate overnight. A few hours before serving, beat egg whites until stiff and fold them gently into the yam mixture. Spoon into individual souffle dishes or a 4-cup (1 litre) large souffle dish sprayed with vegetable oil. Sprinkle tops with a few nuts and a dash of cinnamon. Refrigerate until ready to bake. Bake at 400 degrees F (200 degrees C) for 25 to 30 minutes or until hot and slightly puffed. Serve immediately.

Chocolight Cake

(58 calories per serving)

Yes, in this case, you can have your cake and eat it too! A one-inch (2.5 cm) slice of this delicious chocolate cake has only 58 calories! The recipe comes from friend and fellow cooking enthusiast Barb Watts.

It keeps moist for days. Makes 24 thin slices.

1¼ cups (300 mL) egg whites (about 8)
1 teaspoon (5 mL) cream of tartar
1 cup (250 mL) white sugar
1 teaspoon (5 mL) vanilla
¼ teaspoon (1 mL) almond extract (optional)
¾ cup (180 mL) cake and pastry flour
¼ cup (60 mL) cocoa
1 cup (250 mL) low fat yogurt

Beat egg whites and cream of tartar at high speed until soft peaks form. Gradually add sugar and flavourings, beating constantly until stiff, shiny peaks form. Sift flour and cocoa together then sift a quarter of the mixture over the egg whites and fold in carefully. Gradually add the remaining flour and cocoa in a similar fashion. Fold in yogurt just until mixed. Spoon into an ungreased angel food cake pan and bake at 325 degrees F (160 degrees C) for 45 to 55 minutes or until cake springs back when lightly pressed. Turn upside-down, resting top of pan on an upturned can or bowl to allow air to circulate. When cool, run knife carefully around the cake sides and invert onto a plate. Serve with fresh berries or a little mocha sabayon sauce.

For Summer Entertaining

Salmon Tartare with Black Bread

Grilled Lemon Chicken with Rosemary

Fresh Asparagus
with
Green Peppercorn Dressing

Shredded Zucchini and Carrot Saute

Wholewheat Baguette Bread

Bulgar Wheat Pilaf

Oranges in Sangria

This stylish but casual menu lends itself to a warm summer evening on the patio. It is quick to prepare and pleasantly light, with its accent on citrus: the salmon starter is marinated in lime juice, the main course flavoured with lemon, and oranges round out the dessert course.

Analysis

Serves 4
777 calories per serving
Protein: 22%
Fat: 24%
Carbohydrate: 54%
Sodium: 510 mg
Cholesterol: 92 mg

(Photo following page 92)

Salmon Tartare

(27 calories per serving)

A special treat for sushi lovers, salmon tartare is raw salmon, finely chopped and marinated or ''cooked'' in lime juice, the same method used to prepare scallops for Mexican seviche. I particularly enjoyed the tartare prepared by chef Jacque Pepin when I attended his cooking classes in Toronto, and this recipe includes some of his robust seasonings.

Serves 8 to 10.

1/4 lb (125 grams) boneless, skinless salmon
2 tablespoons (30 mL) lime juice
1 teaspoon (5 mL) grated lime zest
1 teaspoons (5 mL) olive or sunflower oil
1 clove garlic, pressed
2 tablespoons (30 mL) finely chopped purple onion
1/3 cup (60 mL) chopped parsley
Pepper to taste
1 teaspoon (5 mL) each of chopped fresh thyme and tarragon (or good pinches of the same herbs, dried)
Several dashes of Tabasco
1/2 teaspoon (2 mL) Dijon mustard
1/2 teaspoon (2 mL) red wine vinegar
To Garnish: butter lettuce, capers, lemon wedges, finely chopped purple onion.

This dish should be prepared on the morning of serving. If salmon is fresh, wrap and freeze it for a few hours until firm. This will make it easier to chop finely. Place chopped salmon in bowl, add the rest of the ingredients and mix well. Refrigerate for several hours. Serve in a mound on a bed of lettuce along with chopped onion, capers and lemon wedges. Serve the same day with black bread or toast points. If you are counting calories, a serving of black bread will add 63.

Grilled Lemon Chicken with Rosemary

(136 calories per serving)

Chicken breasts pick up a tart citrus flavour from a herbed marinade before cooking on a hot grill. You can try this marinade with limes instead of lemons for an interesting difference. Serves 4.

4 single chicken breasts
zest and juice of 2 lemons or limes
1 teaspoon (5 mL) oil
Pepper to taste
1 teaspoon (5 mL) fresh minced ginger
1 teaspoon (5 mL) Dijon or whole seed mustard
1 teaspoon (5 mL) fresh rosemary, finely chopped or 1/2 teaspoon (2 mL) dried rosemary or tarragon

Debone chicken breasts and remove the skin. Cover and refrigerate while you make the marinade by combining the rest of the ingredients. A few hours before serving time, marinate the chicken in the sauce, keeping it in the refrigerator. Turn over the chicken a few times to coat well.

Brush barbecue grill with oil and bring to high heat. Grill the chicken about 3 to 4 minutes per side, depending on thickness, basting frequently with the marinade. Do not overcook. Serve immediately with wedges of lemon or lime.

This chicken is also good cold for picnics. Serve it with Curry Sauce (see Index).

Fresh Asparagus with Green Peppercorn Dressing

(160 calories per serving)

This is my version of a salad featured at Trumps, one of Los Angeles' outstanding restaurants. The unique and zesty dressing can also be used with a salad of prawns, melon and avocado slices on a bed of butter lettuce.

Serves 4.

2 1/4-inch thick (6 mm) round slices of goat cheese (approx. 1/2 oz (14 g) per serving)
1/2 tablespoon (7 mL) sunflower oil
1/2 cup (125 mL) fresh wholewheat breadcrumbs
24 thin spears of fresh asparagus
For garnish: 20 seedless green grapes, butter lettuce

Early on the day of serving, dip cheese rounds in a little oil, roll in bread-crumbs to coat well and refrigerate. Trim and clean asparagus and steam until cooked, but still slightly crisp. Cool quickly in ice water to keep the colour bright, pat dry and refrigerate. Just before serving, divide asparagus among four lettuce-lined plates and drizzle over some of the dressing. Bake the cheese at 400 degrees F (200 degrees C) for about 5 minutes. Cut each round in half and place a piece on top of the asparagus. Sprinkle each plate with peeled grapes and pass more dressing.

Dressing

1 tablespoon (15 mL) green peppercorns, washed and strained
1 cup (500 mL) green seedless grapes, skins on
3 tablespoons (45 mL) vegetable oil

Combine peppercorns and grapes in food processor and process until creamy. Slowly add oil and blend until thick. Refrigerate, covered, for up to several days ahead. Shake well before use.

Shredded Zucchini and Carrots Saute

(80 calories per serving)

Elizabeth and Rob Lloyd-Smith first served me shredded zucchini cooked this way and I've been making it ever since. It is quick to prepare and very tasty. Here, I grated carrots for extra colour and flavour. For best results, this dish should be sauteed quickly at the last minute. Serves 4.

2 medium zucchini
2 large carrots, peeled
1 large or 2 small cloves of garlic, crushed
Lots of freshly-ground pepper
1 tablespoon (15 mL) butter (or 1 tablespoon chicken stock)

Early on the day of serving, grate the zucchini and carrots separately medium-fine using a food processor or a medium grater. Let vegetables sit for a few minutes, then squeeze them dry in clean tea towels. Mix them together and refrigerate, covered, until ready to serve.

Heat butter in large skillet (or spray with vegetable coating and add chicken stock), saute the garlic, then add the grated vegetables and fry over fairly high heat, stirring constantly for one to two minutes until they are just tender. Serve immediately with lots of pepper.

Bulgar Rice Pilaf

(180 calories per serving)

This combination of cracked wheat bulgar and brown rice spiked with turmeric and lemon gives this dish a unique flavour and nut- like texture. It can be made the day ahead and reheated in the oven or microwave oven Serves 6.

1 teaspoon (5 mL) butter
1/2 cup (125 mL) cracked wheat bulgar
1/2 cup (125 mL) brown rice, washed and strained
1/2 teaspoon (2 mL) turmeric
2 cups (500 mL) plus 3 tablespoons (45 mL) chicken stock
zest and juice of 1/2 lemon

Melt the butter in a skillet over medium heat. Saute the bulgar and rice with the turmeric for a few minutes until they are golden. Add boiling chicken stock and simmer for 25 to 30 minutes until bulgar and rice are tender and all the stock absorbed. Add zest and juice of lemon and toss. Refrigerate, covered, or freeze until needed. Reheat to serve in a regular or microwave oven.

Oranges in Sangria

(125 calories per serving)

Refreshing, colourful and nutritious, a dessert you can drink as well as eat! Serve it with Blackberry Ice for a stunning colour and flavour combination. For best results, make this a day or two ahead. Serves 4.

1 cup (250 mL) freshly squeezed orange juice
2 cups (500 mL) dry red wine
2 tablespoons (30 mL) white sugar
4 large oranges, peeled and all pith removed
2 tablespoons (30 mL) Grand Marnier or other orange liqueur

Make the sangria marinade by combining orange juice, wine and sugar in saucepan. Bring to a boil and simmer until mixture has reduced to 1 1/2 cups (375 mL). Cool. Pour 1 cup (250 mL) of the marinade over the oranges in a bowl and sprinkle them with Grand Marnier. Cover and refrigerate. Baste the oranges with the marinade from time to time.

Add an additional 1 tablespoon (15 mL) white sugar to the remaining 1/2 cup (125 mL) of the marinade and reduce over medium heat until thick and reduced by about half. Cover and store in refrigerator. To serve, place oranges in a glass compote dish, pour the sangria over and around and glaze each orange with the thickened sangria. Serve with Blackberry Ice (see Index) and decorate with strips of orange zest. Provide a knife and fork for eating this, and serve the left-over sangria in glasses.

Coast to Coast Celebration

Prawns with Tropical Dip

Spinach Salad
with Warm Chevre Cheese

Wholewheat Bagel Crisps

Grilled Marinated Fillet of Salmon and Onions

Hot Potato Salad

Multi-Grain Bread

Poached Pears
with Blackberry Ice and Two Sauces

Inspired by the freshness of Canadian seafood, fruits and vegetables, this versatile menu adapts easily to a number of occasions, at home, at the cottage or on the boat. All of the cooked dishes are equally good served hot or cold and this makes it very easy on the hostess. Either the prawns or the salad could be left out for a simpler meal.

Analysis

Serves 8 to 10
911 calories per serving
Protein: 26%
Fat: 29%
Carbohydrate: 45%
Sodium: 460 mg
Cholesterol: 159 mg

(Photo following page 92)

Steamed Prawns with Tropical Dip

(73 calories per serving)

In this dish, it's the dip that raises the eyebrows. Everyone is intrigued by its taste and tries to guess the ingredients. I enjoy serving seafood with fruit and this combination is most interesting. Allow about 2 prawns per serving. Serves 8 to 10.

1 1/2 lbs (.75 kilo) fresh uncooked whole prawns
1/2 cup (125 mL) water, just enough to cover the prawns
1 clove garlic, chopped
1/2 lemon, sliced

Early on the morning of serving, bring the water, lemon slices and garlic to a boil, add prawns and steam, covered, until they just turn pink, only about two minutes. Do not overcook. Strain prawns and leave until cool enough to peel. Leave tails on. Chill until ready to serve.

Tropical Dip

1 banana, ripe but not brown
1 ripe avocado
1 ripe mango or papaya or 2 peaches
Juice and zest of 1 large lime (or to taste)
1 tablespoon (15 mL) pineapple juice

I prefer mango for this. If fresh fruit is not available, substitute canned. Just before serving, put all ingredients into a food processor or blender and blend well.

To serve: spoon dip into bowl and place in centre of large platter. Arrange prawns all around and decorate with limes. Pass cut limes to squeeze on the prawns before dipping.

Spinach Salad with Warm Chevre Cheese

(160 calories per serving)

Goat cheese or chevre is the star cheese of the eighties. It has less fat than most whole milk cheese and is easier to digest. North American brands tend to be more delicate in flavour and less salty than imported varieties. I use Canadian Snow Goat.

This combination of spinach, radicchio and warm goat cheese with a delicate vinaigrette dressing is a winner. It was inspired by the specialty salad of Spago's restaurant in Los Angeles, created by their celebrity chef Wolfgang Puck. Even my friends who swear they don't like goat cheese wolf this salad down. And if you're afraid the name will put them off, simply call it French Cheese Salad, a trick I learned from one of my students who owns a pub.

Serves 6 to 8.

Salad Greens
1 head radicchio or small red cabbage
2 bunches fresh spinach
1/4 cup (60 mL) toasted pine nuts

Clean and dry spinach and separate leaves of radicchio or cabbage. Stack leaves in piles, roll up jelly-roll fashion and cut on the diagonal into thin strips. This is called chiffonade. You should have almost 2 cups (500 mL) of radicchio or cabbage strips and 3 cups (750 mL) of spinach strips. Set greens aside in refrigerator until ready to use.

Dressing

1/2 cup (125 mL) virgin olive oil
3 to 4 tablespoons (45 to 60 mL) balsamic vinegar or red wine vinegar
1/4 teaspoon (1 mL) Dijon mustard
Pepper to taste

Blend well and refrigerate.

Cheese

4 1/4-inch thick (6mm) slices of goat cheese (about 1/2 oz, 14 g per serving)
The cheese comes in small-diameter rolls
1/2 teaspoon (2 mL) virgin olive oil
3/4 cup (180 mL) fresh wholewheat breadcrumbs
1/2 teaspoon (2 mL) each of dried basil, oregano and thyme
(or 1 1/2 teaspoons (7 mL) each of fresh herbs)

Early on the day of serving, combine breadcrumbs and herbs. Roll the goat cheese in a little oil then coat with the herbed crumbs. Refrigerate. Just before serving, bake coated cheese for about 5 minutes at 400 degrees F (200 degrees C) or until golden.

To serve: toss salad greens with enough dressing to coat and arrange on 6 to 8 salad plates. Sprinkle with fresh pepper and a few toasted pinenuts. Cut each round of baked cheese in half and place in the centre of each plate. Serve with bagel crisps.

Wholewheat Bagel Crisps

(21 calories per crisp)

These are marvellous for soups and salads or just for munching. They keep for days in a sealed container. Makes about 24 to 30.

4 wholewheat, plain or pumpernickel day-old bagels
safflower or sunflower oil
3 garlic cloves, peeled and halved

Slice the bagels in very thin horizontal slices. Brush both sides with a little oil and place on large cookie sheet. Spear half a garlic clove on a fork, cut side down, and rub both sides of the bagel slices. Replace clove as it loses its oil. Bake bagel slices at 275 degrees F (135 degrees C) for 60 minutes or until golden and crisp, turning them over at half time. Cool on racks, store in container.

Grilled Marinated Salmon and Onions

(222 calories per serving)

A filleted whole salmon is marinated with just a touch of Oriental flavourings which the onions pick up as they grill to a crispy brown. Serves 8.

1 salmon fillet, skin on, about 2 lbs (1 kilo)
or 2 baby coho salmon, deboned
4 large purple onions, sliced into thirds
1/4 cup (60 mL) soy sauce (low sodium)
1/4 cup (60 mL) dry sherry or sherry vinegar
2 tablespoons (30 mL) rice wine vinegar
2 tablespoons (30 mL) sunflower oil
1 tablespoon (15 mL) sesame oil
3 tablespoons (45 mL) chopped green onion or shallots
1 clove garlic, chopped

Blend together all ingredients except for salmon and onions. About two to three hours before serving, lay the salmon fillet in a large shallow casserole, skin side down. Pour over enough of the marinade to cover and refrigerate. Marinate onion slices at room temperature in the same mixture. Turn salmon and onions once or twice. Reserve leftover marinade for basting.

Oil barbecue grill well and place over high heat (either gas or hot coals). Lay salmon and onions on grill and cook for about 4 to 5 minutes on each side, basting well. Salmon should just be opaque and onions a dark crispy golden. Decorate with lemon wedges and sprigs of cilantro, parsley or fresh dill. Serve hot or cold.

Greek Tsatziki (see Chef on the Run) makes an excellent alternative accompaniment for this salmon dish.

Hot Potato Salad

(158 calories per serving)

This warm salad goes well with any barbecue menu and can also be served cold. Its dressing is spiked with fresh basil. Serves 10 to 12.

8 cups (2 litres) tiny new red potatoes, cooked and cubed
1 cup (250 mL) corn kernels, cooked (fresh or frozen)
1/2 cup (125 mL) finely chopped red pepper
1/2 cup (125 mL) finely chopped yellow pepper
3 medium tomatoes, peeled, seeded and cubed
Pepper to taste

Green pepper can be substituted for red and yellow. Combine all ingredients a day ahead of serving and add enough of the following dressing to coat. Cover and refrigerate. The next morning you might need to add a little more dressing to keep the salad moist. To serve hot, simply heat everything in a heavy skillet until just warm.

Dressing

1 cup (250 mL) fresh basil leaves
or 1/4 cup (60 mL) dried basil
1/4 cup (60 mL) virgin olive oil or sunflower oil
1/2 teaspoon (2 mL) Dijon mustard
4 tablespoons (60 mL) red wine vinegar
5 tablespoons (75 mL) chopped green onions or shallots
Pepper to taste

Combine all ingredients in a blender or food precessor, adding the oil very slowly. This can be made the day ahead of serving.

Poached Pears with Blackberry Ice and Two Sauces

(257 calories per serving)

I fell in love with this dessert one evening at Oliver's, an outstanding restaurant in Toronto. This is my version. A pear poached in wine is served on a plate with two sauces, a raspberry puree and a rich vanilla creme. Then, to gild the lily, I add small scoops of home-made blackberry ice. All the elements of this dessert can be prepared ahead of time. Serves 8.

Poached Pears

(111 calories per serving)

4 pears, ripe but firm (Bosc pears give the best results)
1/2 cup (125 mL) white wine
1/4 cup (60 mL) fructose (fruit sugar)
Juice of 1/2 lemon
Water to cover

Cut pears in half, leaving half the stem on each, and remove core with melon ball cutter. Place pears immediately in a large saucepan with the rest of the ingredients. Bring to a boil and simmer, partially covered, for about 10 minutes or until pears are just tender. Do not overcook. Remove pears. Cool liquid. Place pears in a bowl and cover with liquid. Seal and refrigerate for up to three days. Serve half a pear per person.

Creme Anglaise

(23 calories per serving)

This sauce is rich in egg yolks but it serves 12 to 16 people since only a tablespoon is required per serving.

4 egg yolks, at room temperature
1/4 cup (60 mL) fructose (fruit sugar)
3/4 cup (180 mL) skim milk
1 teaspoon (5 mL) vanilla

A day or two ahead of serving, combine yolks and sugar in a large saucepan and whisk until creamy, about 3 minutes. Add milk in a steady stream. Place over medium heat and cook, stirring constantly with a wooden spoon, until the mixture is thickened and coats the spoon. Watch carefully as it curdles easily. Add vanilla. Cool and refrigerate.

Raspberry Sauce

(11 calories per serving)

Puree 2 small packages raspberries frozen without sugar or 2 cups fresh raspberries until smooth. Pour twice through a fine sieve to remove seeds and refrigerate. For variation, substitute blackberries or strawberries.

Blackberry Ice

(112 calories per serving)

A refreshing, melt-in-the-mouth sorbet. If blackberries are unavailable or you're pressed for time, Hagan-Daas boysenberry ice is good. Serves 6.

4 cups (1 litre) blackberries, fresh or frozen
3/4 cup (180 mL) white sugar
1 1/2 cups (375 mL) water

Slowly heat blackberries, crushing them with a potato masher to release the juices. Strain through a sieve. This should yield 2 cups (500 mL) juice. Boil water and sugar together for 5 to 8 minutes to make a light syrup. Cool. Mix with juice and freeze in shallow pan. When mushy, scrape into a blender and blend until smooth. Refreeze. To serve, take it from freezer to soften slightly and serve in tiny scoops, about 3 tablespoons per serving.

To assemble dessert: On individual dessert plates place about 2 tablespoons (30 mL) of raspberry puree. Add 1 tablespoon (15 mL) of vanilla cream to centre and with a knife tip swirl to blend the sauces slightly. Place pear half in the upper middle of the plate and on either side place tiny scoops of Blackberry Ice. Decorate with a sprig of mint.

The Italian Connection

Marinated Vegetable Platter

Osso Buco with Fettucine

Italian Bread

Melon and Raspberries in Galliano

This hearty Italian dinner is perfect for ''carbo''-loading before a marathon or for hungry guests who just love pasta. The classic Osso Buco is at its best made a day ahead of serving and so is the marinated vegetable platter, a different version of Italian antipasto. Provide plenty of Italian bread to soak up the veal sauce and end the meal with a light fresh fruit compote.

Analysis

Serves 6 to 8
577 calories per serving
Protein: 21%
Fat: 25%
Carbohydrate: 54%
Sodium: 603 mg
Cholesterol: 65 mg

(Photo following page 92)

Marinated Vegetable Platter

(72 calories per serving)

This unusual salad was inspired by a recipe given to me by Julie Elevin on a recent visit to Sydney, Australia. Fresh mushrooms, beets and artichokes marinate overnight in a tart dressing with just a touch of sun-dried tomatoes added at the last minute. It's perfect for a barbecue or a patio dinner party.

Serves 8 to 10.

2 cups (500 mL) medium-size fresh mushrooms, cleaned and thickly sliced
2 cups (500 mL) cooked fresh beets, sliced about 1/4 inch (6 mm) thick
3 14 oz (398 mL) cans whole artichoke hearts, drained (If they are large, cut in half)
4 pickled French style gherkins, chopped
1/3 cup (80 mL) sun-dried tomatoes, sliced in thin strips or chopped (or substitute pimento or red pepper strips)
1/2 cup (125 mL) finely chopped parsley
1 large curly-leaf lettuce, cleaned and dried

Dressing

1 1/2 cups (375 mL) vegetable oil
3 cloves garlic, crushed
6 tablespoons (90 mL) red wine vinegar
4 tablespoons (60 mL) finely chopped green onion or shallots
4 tablespoons (60 mL) finely chopped parsley
1/2 teaspoon (2 mL) Dijon mustard
1/2 teaspoon (2 mL) each dried or 2 teaspoons (10 mL) each fresh oregano, basil, marjoram and thyme
Pepper to taste

Combine all very well in blender or food processor. Refrigerate, covered. This should be made several days ahead.

On the day ahead: Prepare vegetables, put into separate bowls and add enough of the dressing to cover. Marinate overnight in the refrigerator. Reserve enough of the dressing to sprinkle over the salad before serving.

On the morning of serving: drain the vegetables, adding a little chopped parsley to the mushrooms and the chopped gherkins to the artichokes. Arrange a layer of lettuce on a large platter, then place concentric circles of mushrooms and artichoke hearts around a central mound of beets. Drizzle a little of the reserved dressing over and sprinkle with the rest of the parsley and a dash of pepper. Arrange the dried tomato strips over the mushrooms and artichokes. Cover with plastic wrap and refrigerate until ready to serve.

Osso Buco

(358 Calories per serving)

Always a hit, this Italian classic of simmered meaty veal bones rates a gold medal. Reduce the fat content of this dish by trimming all visible fat and by browning the veal in a tiny amount of oil. I always make this dish the day before serving and reheat it — the flavour seems to improve. Any form of pasta or rice goes well with this . I prefer fettucine, either a combination of spinach and white or a lemon pepper variety if you can find one. Serves 8.

1 tablespoon (15 mL) virgin olive oil
1/3 cup (80 mL) wholewheat flour
Pepper
8 veal shanks (about 3 1/2 lbs, 1 3/4 kilos with bone,
yield, about 1 1/4 lbs of meat (1/2 kilo))
1 cup (250 mL) dry white wine
1 cup (250 mL) low-sodium beef bouillon or home-made stock
1 28-oz (796 mL) can Italian plum tomatoes, chopped, with juice
1 yellow or purple onion, chopped
1 yellow and 1 red pepper in julienne strips
(green pepper can be substituted)
4 sticks celery, chopped (equals 1 cup, 250 mL)
3 large carrots, chopped (about 1½ cups, 375 mL)
1 1/2 teaspoons (7 mL) dried basil
or 4 teaspoons (20 mL) fresh basil
1 teaspoon (5 mL) dried oregano
or 3 teaspoons (15 mL) fresh oregano
1 teaspoon (5 mL) dried thyme
or 3 teaspoons (15 mL) fresh thyme

Heat oil in skillet. Roll veal shanks just to coat slightly in the flour and pepper and brown a few at a time. Set aside. To the skillet add the wine and stir to deglaze the pan. Add the rest of the ingredients, bring to a boil and simmer for ten minutes.

Place veal shanks in a large Dutch oven and pour over them the contents of the skillet. Bake at 350 degrees F (180 degrees C) for about 1½ hours, covered, then uncover and bake for a further 30 minutes. Cool, then refrigerate overnight.

Skim off any fat from surface and reheat at 350 degrees F (180 degrees C) for about 30 minutes until hot, or reheat in microwave oven.

Prepare pasta or rice, place in large serving dish and arrange veal on top. Sprinkle with about 4 tablespoons (60 mL) of fresh-grated Parmesan cheese and sprinkle with the following Gremolata: Combine 1 tablespoon (15 mL) grated zest of lemon, 2 pressed cloves of garlic and ½ cup (125 mL) of coarsely chopped parsley. Pass extra Parmesan cheese.

Melon and Raspberries in Galliano

(72 calories per serving)

The Italian liqueur Galliano with its hint of licorice imparts its unique taste to the fruit. Try it also with a combination of fresh peaches and blueberries.

Serves 10 to 12.

2 cantaloupe melons, scooped into small balls with a melon cutter
2 cups (500 mL) fresh raspberries
2 to 3 tablespoons (30 to 45 mL) Galliano

Marinate the fruit separately in the Galliano for about 20 minutes before serving. Refrigerate. Drain and serve, arranging the fruit in alternate layers in individual goblets or a large glass bowl.

California Pizzalina Party

Apple Mulled Wine Soup

Make your own Pizzas

Angel Cake
with Creme Anglaise and Raspberry Puree

This idea for this make-your-own low-cal pizza was inspired by the innovative pizzas featured at Wolfgang Puck's Los Angeles restaurant, Spago's. Ideal for hungry teenagers or for an apres-ski crowd, the pizzas start with a wholewheat crust, prepared in advance. The guests concoct their own toppings from an assortment of vegetables, cheeses and seafoods and a delicious home-made tomato sauce. The mulled wine soup makes an unusual starter and the dessert has far fewer calories than its festive look suggests.

Analysis

(Combination of 4 pizzas, allowing a total of two pizzas per person)

Serves 6
1469 calories per serving
Protein: 20%
Fat: 25%
Carbohydrate: 55%
Sodium 3570 mg
Cholesterol: 134 mg

(Photo following page 124)

Apple Mulled Wine Soup

(158 calories per serving)

Made a day ahead, its mulled wine base enhanced by apples and cranberry juice, this soup is served in mugs, perfect for the apres-ski crowd.

Serves 6 to 8.

3 cups (750 mL) boiling water
2 tablespoons (30 mL) honey or fructose
6 tart, green apples (Granny Smith or Newton)
1 cinnamon stick
zest of 1 lemon
1 teaspoon (5 mL) vanilla
1 tablespoon (15 mL) cornstarch
2 tablespoons (30 mL) cranberry juice
Juice of 1 lemon
2 tablespoons (30 mL) red or blackcurrant jelly
1/4 cup (60 mL) cranberry juice
2 cups (500 mL) dry red wine

Peel, core and slice the apples. In a large saucepan, combine water, honey, cinnamon stick, lemon zest and vanilla and simmer for about 15 minutes until apples are just tender. Puree until smooth. Dissolve cornstarch in the 2 tablespoons (30 mL) of cranberry juice and add to the puree along with all the rest of the ingredients. Simmer for 10 minutes. Add a pinch of freshly grated nutmeg. Cool and refrigerate overnight.

To serve: reheat until almost boiling and ladle into mugs, allowing about 1/2 cup (125 mL) per person. Top with a dollop of yogurt, a sprinkle of nutmeg and a cinnamon stick.

Pizzalina

A pizza that's leaner — lower in calories — and with a wholesome, crisp wholewheat crust. I've suggested four California-style toppings, mostly with a home-made tomato sauce base, but it's fun to try other combinations. Teenagers are particularly good at this. Just put out an assortment of good things and watch them go to work! They also make great appetizers: make them ahead of time and reheat for 5 to 8 minutes at 350 degrees F (180 degrees C) or until hot.

Pizza Crust

(520 calories per serving, 2 pizzas)

2 tablespoons (30 mL) instant yeast
2 teaspoons (10 mL) honey
4 tablespoons (60 mL) vegetable oil
5 to 6 cups (1250 to 1500 mL) wholewheat flour
2 cups (500 mL) warm water
cornmeal for the cookie sheet

Dissolve the yeast and honey in the warm water, add oil and stir to mix. Let stand for a few minutes. Put 5 cups (1250 mL) flour into a food processor, pour in the liquid and mix until it forms soft ball. Add the rest of the flour if dough is too soft. Knead for a few minutes on a floured board. If mixing by hand, stir into the yeast mixture about half the flour, beating well with wooden spoon. Knead in rest of flour by hand.

Put dough into a medium-sized bowl sprayed with vegetable oil coating, cover with a damp cloth and leave in a warm place to rise for about 1 hour or until doubled. Punch down and form into a long roll. Divide roll into 12 equal pieces. (The dough can be frozen at this stage, if desired. Thaw before completing.) Roll each piece out into a 6-inch (15-cm) round of about 1/8-inch (3 mm) thickness, forming a thicker rim around the edges. Brush with a little oil and arrange the toppings to your liking. Place pizzas on large cookie sheet lined with cornmeal and bake at 500 degrees F (250 degrees C) for 10 to 12 minutes or until crust is crisp and cheese melted.

Tomato Sauce for Pizzas

(114 calories per serving, 2 pizzas)

2 cups (500 mL) tomato coulis (see index)
6 tablespoons (90 mL) tomato paste
2 cloves of garlic, crushed

Combine all ingredients, bring to a boil and simmer for about 10 minutes. Cool. Makes enough sauce for 12 6-inch pizzas. Freezes well.

Spread 3 tablespoons (45 mL) of the tomato sauce over each pizza as a base for the following combinations:

Seafood Pizza

(220 calories per pizza, topping only)

Prawns, scallops or other seafood, cooked
artichoke hearts, chopped
Sun-dried tomatoes, thinly sliced
Goat cheese, 1 tablespoon (15 mL) per pizza
Parmesan cheese

Arrange ingredients decoratively over the tomato sauce-covered pizza, dotting on tiny dabs of goat cheese and topping everything with freshly-grated Parmesan cheese.

Pizza Primavera

(195 calories per pizza, topping only)

Thin slices tomatoes
Thin slices zucchini
Thin slices purple onion
Thin slices mushrooms
Shredded fontina cheese, 1 tablespoon (15 mL) per pizza
Grated Parmesan cheese, 2 teaspoons (10 mL) per pizza
Pinches of basil and oregano

Circle tomato slices on tomato-sauce base and top with the suggested vegetables in layers. Top with the cheese and herbs.

Prosciutto and Cantaloupe

(276 calories per pizza, topping only)

Several pieces of goat cheese, enough to cover pizza
Thin strips of prosciutto ham
Finely chopped shallots or green onion
Cubed cantaloupe
Chopped Parsley

Sprinkle a thin layer of goat cheese over the tomato sauce base and sprinkle with shallots or onions. Bake for 10 to 15 minutes until crust is crisp and cheese melted. Top with the ham and cantaloupe and return to oven for a few minutes to heat through. Top with parsley.

Smoked Salmon Pizza

(190 calories per pizza, topping only)

Goat cheese
Sliced purple onion
Thin slices of smoked salmon
Dill, fresh or dried
Capers, optional

Put a thin layer of the goat cheese directly on the pizza crust (no tomato sauce). Sprinkle over a layer of purple onion and bake for about 10 minutes. Add salmon and dill and a little more goat cheese and return to oven to heat through. Just before serving, add more salmon and raw onion and capers if you are using them.

Jennifer's Angel Food Cake, with Creme Anglaise and Raspberry Puree

(193 calories per serving)

Angel food cake, first launched in the 1950s, is enjoying a modest revival. Requiring no egg yolks and a perfect complement to fresh fruit, it's very definitely food for the 80s. Here it is served with Creme Anglaise and Raspberry Puree (see Index) for a beautiful presentation. The recipe itself comes from my mother's collection, and it is our daughter Jennifer's favourite.

Note: for a high and light cake, it is important to sift the flour with half the sugar three or four times. The tube pan should not be greased.

Serves 12 to 14.

1 cup (250 mL) sifted cake flour
3/4 cup (180 mL) fine granulated or berry sugar
1 1/2 cups (375 mL) egg whites (about 12 large)
1 1/2 teaspoons (7 mL) cream of tartar
1/4 teaspoon (1 mL) salt
1 1/2 teaspoons (7 mL) vanilla
3/4 cup (180 mL) fine granulated or berry sugar.

Sift flour with the 3/4 cup (180 mL) sugar three or four times. Beat egg whites, cream of tartar and vanilla until mixture is stiff but still moist and shiny. Slowly add the remaining sugar, about a tablespoon (15 mL) at a time, beating all the while. Sift about 1/4 of the flour over the whites and fold in lightly with a down-up-over motion while turning the bowl. Add the remaining flour gradually, continuing to fold in lightly. Pile mixture carefully into a 10-inch (25 cm) tube pan, making sure there are no air pockets.

Bake for about 40 to 45 minutes at 350 degrees F (180 degrees C) or until cake springs back when touched. Invert pan and cool. Angel cake freezes beautifully.

To serve: On individual large white plates place a pool of Creme Anglaise on one side, a pool of Raspberry Puree on the other. (See Index for recipes). Place a piece of cake in the centre and decorate with sliced strawberries, fresh raspberries, melon balls or other fruit in season.

Fuel Foods

Corn Chips with Salsa

Harvest Vegetable Basket

Yogurt Dip

Black Bean Soup

Graham Bread

Baked Stuffed Cinnamon Apples

Carob Crispies

This menu for eight is guaranteed to give you energy plus! It's healthy, satisfying food, perfect for a hungry family on a cold winter's night, or for weekends at the ski cabin. The fresh vegetables, bread and baked apples provide an abundance of vitamins, minerals and fibre and the bean soup is rich in protein. The yogurt dip and topping give calcium for an overall high nutrition count.

Analysis

Serves 8
1272 calories per serving
Protein: 16%
Fat: 22%
Carbohydrate: 62%
Sodium: 271 mg
Cholesterol: 20 mg

(Photo following page 124)

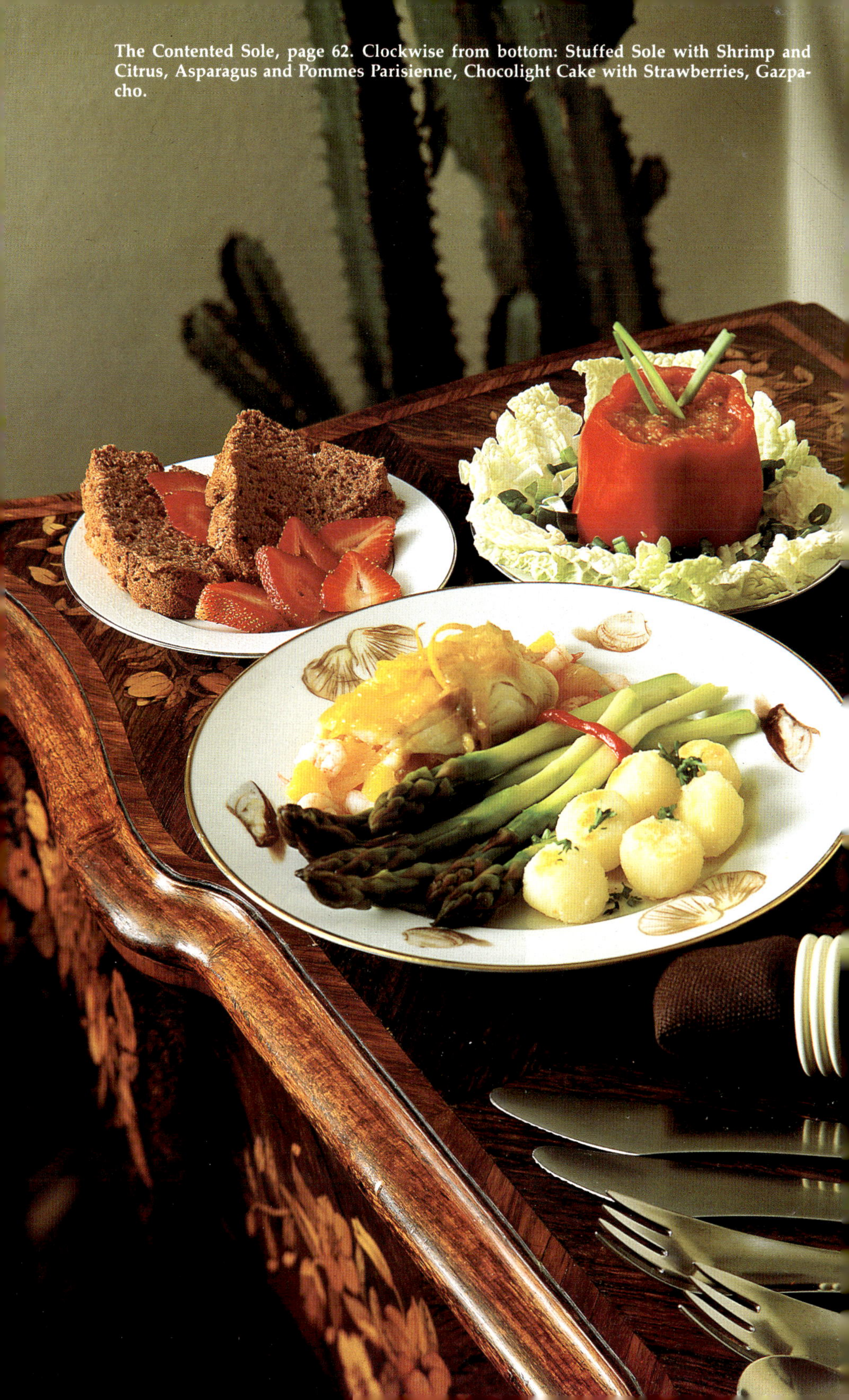

The Contented Sole, page 62. Clockwise from bottom: Stuffed Sole with Shrimp and Citrus, Asparagus and Pommes Parisienne, Chocolight Cake with Strawberries, Gazpacho.

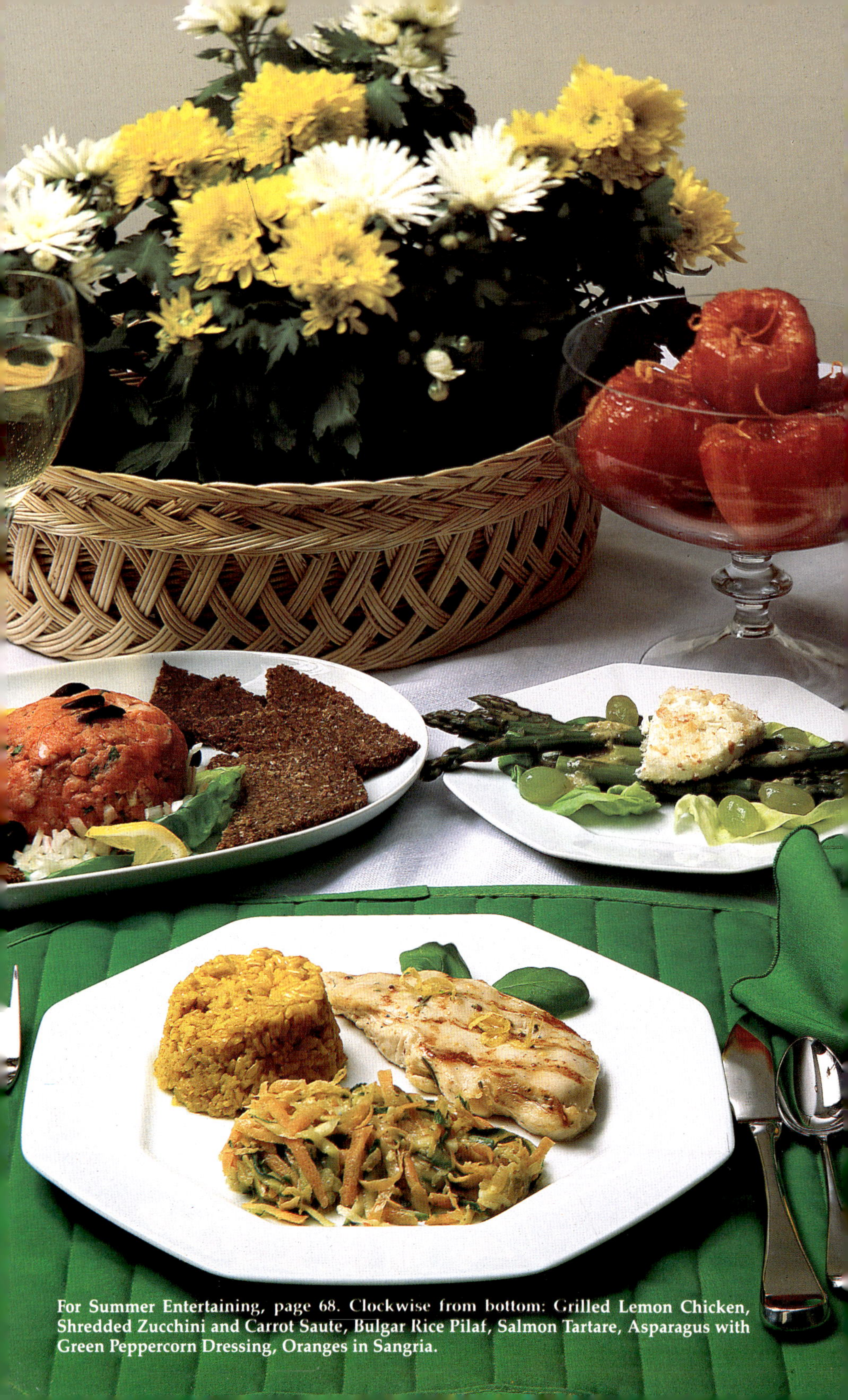

For Summer Entertaining, page 68. Clockwise from bottom: Grilled Lemon Chicken, Shredded Zucchini and Carrot Saute, Bulgar Rice Pilaf, Salmon Tartare, Asparagus with Green Peppercorn Dressing, Oranges in Sangria.

Coast to Coast Celebration, page 74. Clockwise from bottom right: Hot Potato Salad, Spinach Salad with Chevre, Poached Pear with Blackberry Ice and Two Sauces, Grilled Salmon and Onions, Prawns with Tropical Dip.

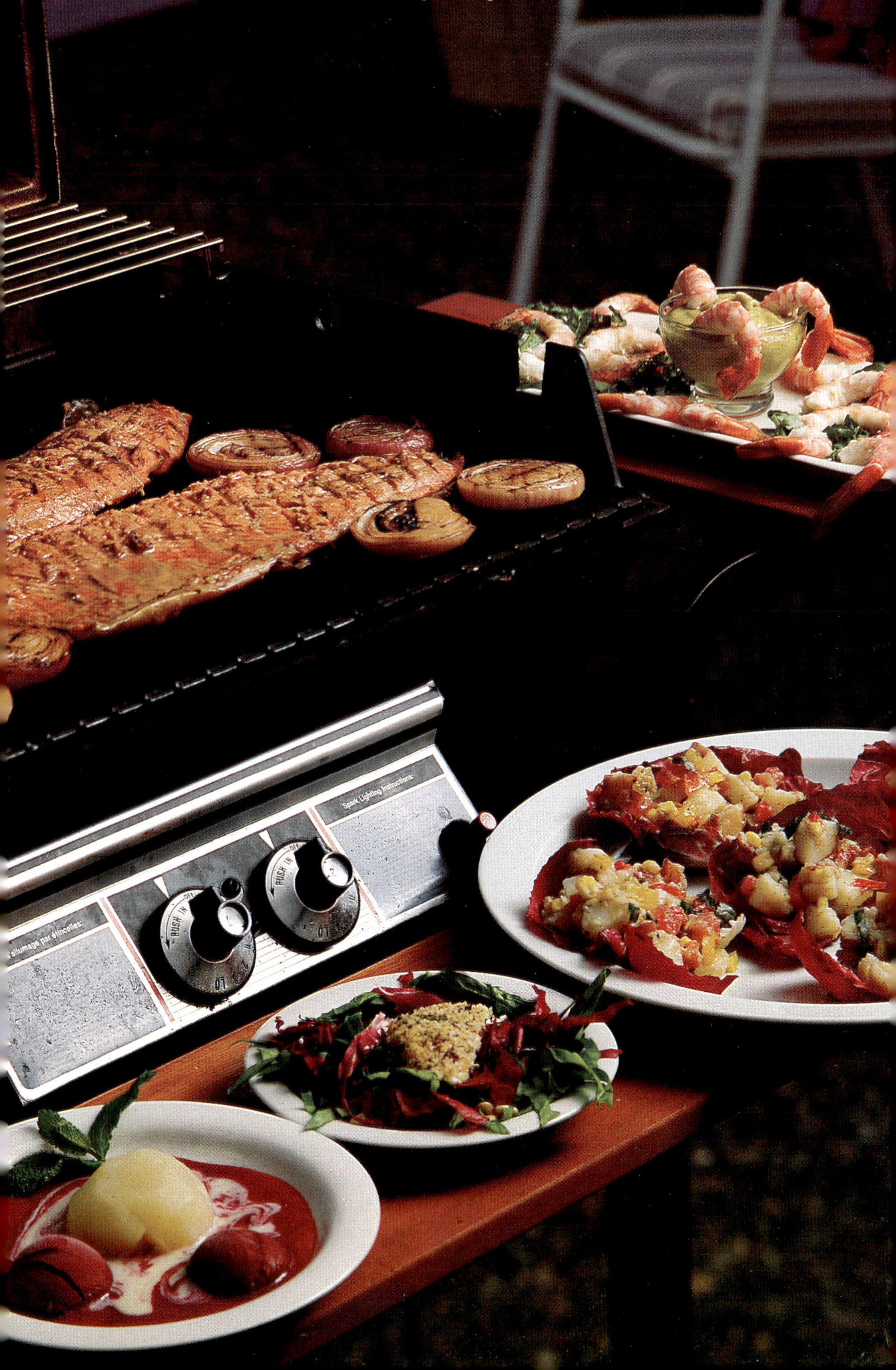

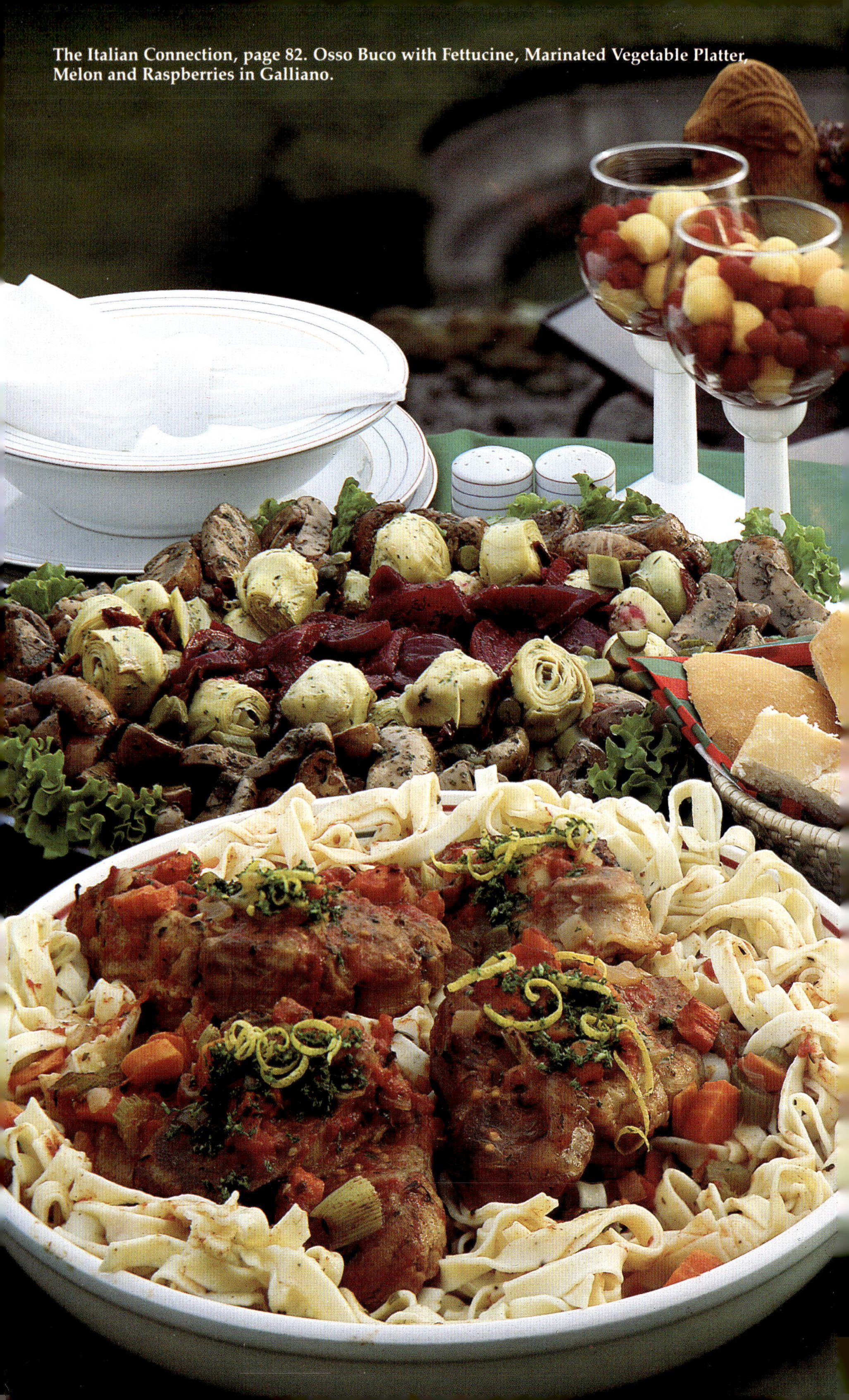

The Italian Connection, page 82. Osso Buco with Fettucine, Marinated Vegetable Platter, Melon and Raspberries in Galliano.

Salsa

(10 calories per serving)

Everyone enjoys dipping hot corn chips into Mexican salsa. Buy natural unsalted corn chips and warm them briefly in the oven before serving. The salsa can be made up several days in advance. Serve it, too, as a topping on the black bean soup — it's marvellous! The specialty ingredients for this recipe can be found in the Mexican food section of your supermarket. (Corn chips add about 150 calories per serving.) Makes about 2 cups (500 mL), to serve 12 to 16.

2 to 3 large ripe tomatoes, finely chopped
About 3 oz (85 g) canned green chilies, finely chopped
1/2 cup (125 mL) canned tomatoes with chilies
2 tablespoons (30 mL) mild or medium taco sauce
2 tablespoons (30 mL) chopped green onion
1 tablespoon (15 mL) red wine vinegar
1 clove garlic, pressed
1/4 teaspoon (1 mL) ground cumin seed
Zest and juice of half a lime
Pepper to taste

Combine all ingredients in food processor or blender, mixing until slightly thick but still coarse. Store in covered container in the refrigerator for up to a week. If you want a hotter dip, add a couple of dashes of tabasco sauce.

Harvest Vegetable Basket with Yogurt Dip

(61 calories per serving)

This magnificent cornucopia of goodness starts with a large wicker basket lined with curly lettuce. Raw or slightly cooked vegetables then fill the basket to overflowing, accompanied by a tangy yogurt dip served up inside a red pepper. Select whatever vegetables are fresh at your market, choosing for colour and texture as well as flavour. I used:

whole mushrooms, cleaned
cherry tomatoes
celery sticks
broccoli spears, steamed to slightly tender
fresh asparagus, steamed to slightly tender
carrots, scrubbed and cut into chunks
purple onion, sliced into rings
jicama (tuber used commonly in Mexican cooking), peeled and cut into thin sticks
daikon (Oriental white radish), peeled and cut into strips
Belgian endive, optional

Yogurt Dip

This is great for dipping the vegetables or with grilled chicken or seafood, or as a salad dressing. Truly versatile. Serves 8.

1/2 cup (125 mL) 2% yogurt, strained overnight in cheesecloth
3/4 cup (180 mL) low-fat ricotta cheese
1 teaspoon (5 mL) Dijon mustard
1 teaspoon (5 mL) red wine vinegar
1 tablespoon (15 mL) finely chopped shallots
2 tablespoons (30 mL) finely chopped green onion
1 clove garlic, pressed
1/4 teaspoon (1 mL) Hungarian sweet paprika
1/4 teaspoon (1 mL) each of dried marjoram and thyme (or 3/4 teaspoon (3 mL) each of fresh herbs)
1/8 teaspoon (.5 mL) Worcestershire sauce
Pepper to taste

Combine all ingredients, whisking with wire whip until creamy. Adjust seasonings and herbs to taste. Store covered in the refrigerator for up to one week. Shake before using. Serve in hollowed out red pepper or red cabbage.

Graham Bread

(120 calories per slice)

This recipe will become one of your classics. It has long been one of mine. I've been baking this loaf for 25 years and it still ranks number one with my family. What's more, it's nutritious. It will keep fresh and moist for several days and freezes very well. I bake it in an 8-cup (2 litre) shortening tin or a large fruit juice can. Makes 1 loaf (16 slices).

2 cups (500 mL) Graham flour
1 cup (250 mL) unbleached white flour
1 tablespoon (15 mL) baking powder
1/2 teaspoon (2 mL) baking soda
Pinch of salt
1 tablespoon (15 mL) brown sugar
2/3 cup (160 mL) skim milk powder
1 3/4 cups (430 mL) water

Mix all dry ingredients together in a medium size bowl. Pour in water and mix by hand, just to blend. Don't overmix. Pour into a well-greased large shortening or juice can, seal top with piece of foil brushed with a little butter and bake at 350 degrees F (180 degrees C) for 1½ hours. Don't peek! Remove from oven and immediately turn out of the tin. The bread is done if it sounds hollow when you tap on the bottom. Cool, wrap in foil and freeze or keep in the refrigerator for up to 3 days. To serve warm, reheat in foil for 10 minutes in a medium oven. This bread makes scrumptious toast.

Black (Turtle) Bean Soup

(595 calories per serving)

Black or turtle beans are a staple food of Latin America and can be found in most health food stores. The soup is thick and hearty and freezes well so it can be made weeks in advance. If serving it fresh, make it two to three days ahead for best flavour. Serve it with a selection of condiments such as Mexican salsa, lemon wedges, chopped red or green peppers, green onions, low-fat yogurt and chopped cilantro or parsley. There's a lot of garlic, but the flavour is perfect for the beans. Serves 8 well.

5 cups (1¼ litres) Mexican black beans, rinsed in cold water
12 cups (3 litres) water
4 cups (1 litre) mild chicken stock
6 cloves garlic, finely chopped
1 bay leaf
1 red pepper, finely chopped
2 small fennel bulbs, finely chopped (1 cup, 250 mL) or 4 stalks celery, finely chopped
1 medium white onion, finely chopped
2 leeks, white only, chopped
3 medium carrots, finely chopped
1½ tablespoons (22 mL) ground cumin seed
1½ tablespoons (22 mL) dried oregano
Pepper to taste
A few shots of Tabasco sauce
½ cup (125 mL) Mexican salsa or mild taco sauce
⅓ cup (80 mL) sherry or dark rum (optional)

Bring water to the boil in a large Dutch oven, add beans and boil for about 5 minutes. Remove from heat and let them steep, covered, for about 90 minutes. Add the rest of the ingredients except for the sherry or rum and continue to simmer for about 1 to 1½ hours, stirring frequently and skimming off the scum. Take out bay leaf, add more stock if you feel it's getting too thick and continue to cook for about another hour or until beans are tender. Stir from time to time. Add sherry or rum.

Take out 3 cups (750 mL) of the soup and puree in processor or blender. Return to the soup and stir well. Freeze in well sealed containers or store in refrigerator. Reheat and serve along with an assortment of condiments.

Baked Stuffed Apples

(191 calories per serving)

There is something comforting about baked apples warm from the oven. However, we must learn to resist the habit of slathering them with whipped cream or ice cream. To satisfy this urge for creaminess, I stuff the apples with a filling that is creamy but with far less sugar and fat than traditional toppings. The apples can be made the day ahead and are equally good hot or cold. Serves 8.

8 medium size Spartan or Granny Smith apples
2 tablespoons (30 mL) cinnamon
2 teaspoons (10 mL) freshly grated nutmeg
3 tablespoons (45 mL) brown sugar
2/3 cup (160 mL) apple juice
1/3 cup (80 mL) orange juice
1/2 teaspoon (2 mL) vanilla

Filling

1 1/2 cups (375 mL) low-fat ricotta cheese
1/4 teaspoon (1 mL) cinnamon
1/2 teaspoon (2 mL) vanilla
1/4 cup (60 mL) fructose
1 tablespoon (15 mL) white or dark rum (optional)
Zest of 1 orange Zest of 1 lemon

A day or two before serving, peel and core the apples. Blend cinnamon, nutmeg and brown sugar and roll apples in the mixture to coat. Spray a shallow casserole with non-stick coating and place apples in pan. Sprinkle any remaining cinnamon mixture in the centre of the apples. Combine apple and orange juices and pour into the pan. Bake in a 400 degree F (200 degree C) oven for 55 to 60 minutes or until just tender basting several times with the juices. Add additional juice if required. Remove apples from oven and cool thoroughly, then cut out some of the apple heart, leaving a solid shell to hold the filling.

Blanch orange and lemon zest in boiling water for 30 seconds, then chop finely. Combine all filling ingredients along with the chopped up pulp from the apples and stuff into the apple centres, dividing the mixture evenly. Chill. To serve, heat, covered for about 15 minutes in a medium oven just until warm. Serve with a dollop of vanilla yogurt.

Carob Crispies

(141 calories per cookie)

Crisp and chunky cookies for a special treat. Carob is an acceptable substitute for chocolate, with far less fat and far more nutrients. It is the ground pod of the honey locust tree and is high in potassium, calcium and phosphorus. You can buy carob chips from a health food store. The cookie mixture is high in calories, so bake them small. Makes 3 1/2 to 4 dozen, depending on size.

1 cup (250 mL) vegetable margarine
3/4 cup (180 mL) brown sugar
1/4 cup (60 mL) boiling water
1 teaspoon (5 mL)) baking soda
1 teaspoon (5 mL) vanilla
2 cups (500 mL) unbleached white flour
1 1/2 cups (375 mL) rolled oats
1/2 cup (125 mL) unsweetened grated coconut
2 cups (500 mL) dark carob chips
1 cup (250 mL) chopped walnuts or pecans

Cream margarine and sugar until light. Add baking soda to boiling water and stir until it stops fizzing. Add vanilla. Pour the vanilla liquid into the creamed mixture and blend well. Mix together the flour, coconut and oats and add to the creamed mixture, blending well. Add chips and walnuts. Form into small balls with your hands and place well apart on a baking sheet lined with foil. Flatten each ball with the palm of the hand until nice and round and flat. Bake at 325 degrees F (160 degrees C) for 15 to 20 minutes until medium brown and toasty. Cool slightly, then remove to cooling racks. Store in airtight containers. They freeze well.

The Flavours of India

Oranges with Fennel and Red Onions

Chicken and Prawn Curry

Basmati Rice

Condiments:
Bananas in Toasted Coconut
Toasted Almonds
Raisins in Port
Fruit Chutney

Chapatis and Poppadums

Pineapple-Orange Sorbet
with Fresh Strawberries

I served this menu on Christmas Eve as a pleasant change of pace from traditional holiday fare. It is great for entertaining on busy days as everything can be prepared in advance, and it lends itself to buffet presentations. I have suggested several condiments to serve with the curry, including a fresh peach chutney that you can make on the day of serving. Ready-made chutneys of various flavours are readily available and can be substituted. The clean, tangy flavour of pineapple makes the sorbet top choice for a perfect ending.

Analysis

Serves 6 to 8
728 calories per serving
Protein: 17%
Fat: 16%
Carbohydrate: 67%
Sodium: 319.6 mg
Cholesterol: 86.6 mg

(Photo following page 124)

Oranges with Fennel and Red Onions

(71 calories per serving)

Although salads are not traditionally served with Indian cuisine, I think this unusual combination works well, served either before or after the curry dish. The spicy dressing is refreshing. Serves 6 to 8.

5 large navel oranges
2 bulbs of fennel
1 large red onion
1 large head of curly endive or leaf lettuce, cleaned and dried.

Marinade

Juice of 2 oranges and 2 lemons
Grated zest of 1 orange and 1 lemon
1/4 teaspoon (1 mL) allspice
1/4 teaspoon (1 mL) cinnamon
1 teaspoon (5 mL) honey

Bring marinade ingredients to a boil, cool, then refrigerate overnight. A few hours before serving, peel oranges, removing all the white pith, and slice crosswise into thin discs. Chill well. Cut off the root and upper leaves of the fennel bulb and discard any brown outer layers. Slice the bulb hearts into thin julienne strips and cover with ice water to crisp for one to two hours. Peel and slice onion paper thin and also keep in ice water.

Line a large platter with the clean lettuce greens and overlap oranges in a circle around the perimeter. Dry onion slices and arrange in a circle inside the oranges, then fill the centre with the drained and dried fennel strips. Shake marinade to mix well and sprinkle over evenly. At this stage the salad platter can be covered with plastic wrap and refrigerated for an hour or so. For a more pungent flavour, steep oranges in the marinade overnight.

Chicken and Prawn Curry

(214 calories per serving)

This exotic curry dish is lower in calories because yogurt replaces the traditional heavy sweet or sour cream. The hot curry spices are balanced with a subtle blend of chutney, lime and mangoes for added flavour. This dish lends itself to different occasions: it can be made the day ahead or at the last minute and reheats beautifully in a regular or microwave oven.

Serves 6 to 8.

1 cup (250 mL) mango chutney (I use Bolst's)
Juice and zest of 1 large or 2 small limes
2 teaspoons (10 mL) curry powder (adjust for personal taste)
2 tablespoons (30 mL) cornstarch
dissolved in 3 tablespoons (45 mL) dry white wine or chicken stock
3 tablespoons (45 mL) chevre cheese or reduced calorie mayonnaise
2 cups (500 mL) plain whole-milk yogurt
1 cup (250 mL) 2% yogurt
2 cups (500 mL) cooked chicken in 1/2 inch (12 mm) cubes
1 large or 2 small fresh mangoes, sliced
or 1 14-oz (398 mL) can sliced mangoes
8 oz (250 grams) cooked, peeled prawns
(If prawns are not desired or unavailable, substitute more chicken)

Combine chutney, lime juice and zest, curry powder and dissolved cornstarch, blend well and bring to a boil in a medium-sized skillet. Simmer for a few minutes until smooth and thickened. Add cheese or mayonnaise, yogurt and chicken and simmer gently for about 25 minutes. At this stage the dish can be cooled and refrigerated.

Just before serving, reheat curry in a 350 degree F oven (180 degrees C) for about 30 minutes, or microwave until heated through. Add sliced mangoes and prawns and heat through. If sauce seems too thick, add more yogurt or a dash of white wine.

Basmati Rice

(181 calories per serving)

An aromatic long grain rice from India, basmati is available at most health food or specialty stores. Rinse thoroughly in strainer before use.

Serves 6 to 8.

2 cups (500 mL) white basmati rice
4 cups (1 litre) Chinese or lemon-scented tea
Juice and zest of 1 lemon

Bring tea to a boil, add rice and simmer, covered, for about 25 minutes until all liquid has been absorbed. Add lemon juice and zest, toss and serve. If necessary, the rice can be made the day ahead and reheated in a medium oven for about 30 minutes or in a microwave oven.

Condiments

Bananas in Coconut: Toast 1 cup (250 mL) of unsweetened, medium-thread coconut in a 350 degree F (180 degree C) oven for about 7 minutes or until golden. This can be made ahead and kept in a sealed jar. Just before serving, peel 2 to 3 ripe bananas, slice thinly and roll them in the coconut. (56 calories per serving).

Toasted Almonds: Toast 1½ cups (375 mL) slivered almonds as above until golden. Make ahead and store in sealed jar. (68 calories per tablespoon).

Raisins in Port: Soak 1½ cups (375 mL) golden raisins in a sealable container with enough port to cover and store in the refrigerator for at least a day. Drain before serving. (40 calories per tablespoon).

Peach Chutney: This is fresh, tart and delicious and can also be made a day or so ahead and kept in the refrigerator. Peel, dice and combine 5 fresh peaches or nectarines (or a combination) with 1 teaspoon (5 mL) honey, 2 tablespoons (30 mL) preserved stem ginger, finely chopped, juice and zest of 2 limes and 3 tablespoons (45 mL) raspberry or blueberry vinegar. If desired, add 1 to 2 tablespoons (15 to 30 mL) of sweet lime chutney, finely chopped. (13 calories per tablespoon).

This is excellent with grilled chicken or seafood.

Pineapple-Orange Sorbet

(85 calories per serving)

Totally refreshing, yet simple to make, this tangy sorbet can be prepared a day ahead. Serves 6 to 8.

2 large ripe pineapples
1 cup (250 mL) fresh orange juice
1 teaspoon (5 mL) honey or fructose
Zest of 1 large orange
2 tablespoons (30 mL) Grand Marnier or other orange liqueur (optional)
2 to $2^1/_2$ cups (500 to 625 mL) fresh strawberries

A day ahead of serving or early the same morning, peel, core and puree the pineapples. They should yield about 4 cups (1 litre). Soak orange zest in boiling water for 1 minute to soften, drain, chop and set aside. Combine pineapple, orange juice and honey and puree in blender or food processor. Strain through a fine sieve and add Grand Marnier. Place in large shallow dish (it should fill only to $^1/_4$ inch (6 mm) deep) and freeze until solid. Puree in food processor until thick and creamy in texture, about 3 to 4 minutes. Pack into shallow dish and freeze again, sealed well.

To serve: Completely line an attractive glass bowl with very thinly sliced strawberries. Scoop out the sorbet and mound in the centre of the strawberries. Decorate with a sprig of fresh mint and serve immediately.

Sunday Brunch

Strawberries 'n Champagne Soup

Giant Dutch Baby Pancake

Fresh Fruit Platter with Yogurt

Apple Carrot Bran Muffins

Juices — Tea — Coffee

This must be my family's favourite Sunday Brunch. After our run (usually around the Stanley Park seawall), we relax for a while reading the Sunday paper before sitting down to a hearty noon breakfast. Yes, the pancake uses eggs but if you cut them out during the rest of the week, you can afford to splurge on Sundays. We serve plenty of fresh fruit alongside the pancake plus a basket of hot muffins and everyone's satisfied. If we are sharing our Sunday Brunch with friends, then the strawberry champagne starter provides a festive touch.

I have the fruit ready, the muffins made, the ingredients for the Dutch Baby measured and the table set before we leave for our run. Then when family and friends are sipping the soup, I whip up the pancake and pop it in the oven. The muffins can be warmed at the last minute. And if the gang is especially hungry, it's easy to whip up a second pancake.

Analysis

Serves 6
755 calories per serving
Protein: 12%
Fat: 25%
Carbohydrate: 63%
Sodium: 310 mg
Cholesterol: 28 mg

(Photo following page 124)

Strawberries 'n Champagne Soup

(82 calories per serving)

When the strawberry season is at its peak, try this delightfully refreshing sparkling chilled soup. The berries must be sweet and juicy. Serves 6.

3 cups (750 mL) strawberries
1/2 cup (125mL) approx. sparkling wine or champagne
To garnish: honey yogurt and fresh mint

Puree the strawberries well, strain and chill. Store in refrigerator. Just before serving, add enough champagne to give the strawberries a tang without making the mixture too thin. Serve in individual glass bowls embedded in larger bowls of crushed ice and garnish each with a dollop of strained, honey-sweetened or plain yogurt and a sprig of mint. Servings should be small — about 1/3 to 1/2 cup (80 to 125 mL).

Giant Dutch Baby Pancake

(300 calories per serving)

The classic Dutch Baby recipe calls for a considerable amount of butter and cream. This version uses butter only sparingly and substitutes skim milk. I make it in my paella pan which is big (16-inch, 40-cm diameter), shallow and holds about 4 quarts (4 litres) of liquid, but it can be made just as well in two smaller skillets provided they are shallow and ovenproof. Serves 6.

1/4 cup (60 mL) butter or margarine, melted
6 eggs
1 1/2 cups (375 mL) skim milk
1 teaspoon (5 mL) vanilla
1 1/2 cups (375 mL) all-purpose unbleached flour

Heat oven to 425 degrees F (220 degrees C). Pour butter or margarine into large pan or smaller skillets and place them in the oven. In a food processor or blender whip eggs together for a few minutes, then add milk and vanilla, then the flour, a little at a time, blending continuously until mixture is smooth. Don't overbeat. Pour batter into the pans and bake on bottom shelf for about 10 to 15 minutes; add warmed apple sauce (see below) spread in an even layer and continue cooking for another 10 minutes or until puffy and golden brown or leave plain and pass the apple separately.

The pancake will collapse a little as soon as you bring it out of the oven so serve it immediately, cut into wedges with a little sprinkle of nutmeg, cinnamon and icing sugar. Let your guests add a dollop of yogurt and help themselves from the fruit platter.

For a change, make the pancake with thin slices of bananas layered on the batter before baking. It's also great with strawberries and yogurt.

Dutch Baby Apple Sauce

4 cups (1 litre) thinly sliced green apples
1 tablespoon (15 mL) apple juice
1 tablespoon (15 mL) brown sugar
1/4 teaspoon (1 mL) cinnamon
1/8 teaspoon (.5 mL) nutmeg
1 tablespoon (15 mL) light rum (optional)

Mix all together in large saucepan and cook gently until apples are soft. Set aside. Serve separately or spread on pancake during baking.

Apple Carrot Bran Muffins

(220 calories per muffin)

One of these muffins will give us many of the nutrients we need every day. They stay moist and fresh for days — the secret of a good muffin recipe. These are high in potassium, phosphorus and Vitamin A. Makes 18 medium or 12 jumbo muffins.

2 eggs
1/2 cup (125 mL) brown sugar
3/4 cup (180 mL) sunflower oil
2 cups (500mL) skim milk
1 cup (250 mL) grated green apple
1 cup (250 mL) grated carrot
1 cup (250 mL) raisins
1 cup (250 mL) bran
1 cup (250 mL) wholewheat flour
1 cup (250 mL) unbleached flour
½ cup (125 mL) wheatgerm
2 teaspoons (10 mL) each of baking soda and baking powder
1/2 tablespoon (7 mL) cinnamon
Apricot or prune halves

Beat eggs lightly; add sugar, oil, milk, apple, carrots and raisins and stir to mix. Combine rest of ingredients and stir in. Cover and chill mixture for at least one hour, preferably overnight. Stir briefly before baking at 375 degrees F (190 degrees C) for about 20 minutes or until done. Serve hot.

These muffins freeze well. Vary the taste by substituting blueberries for the raisins, or chopped dates for the carrots and top each one with apricots or prunes for variety.

The Basics

Chicken Stock

(30 calories per cup)

Canned chicken stock and bouillon cubes are generally high in sodium. Besides, once you taste the difference that home-made stock can make, you will never again want to use them. Make a double batch of this stock: it freezes well. Makes about 6 cups (1.5 litres).

About 4 lbs (2 kilos) of chicken backs, necks, wings
12 cups (3 litres) boiling water
2 large onions studded with three cloves
3 leeks, white parts only, chopped
1 clove garlic, chopped
4 stalks of celery, chopped
1/2 cup (125 mL) chopped parsley
Small bay leaf
Pepper to taste
3 sprigs each of fresh thyme and rosemary or good pinches of dried herbs

Put all the ingredients into a large stock pot or Dutch oven and bring to a boil, removing the froth and scum that rises to the top several times. Simmer for 3 hours uncovered, adding more water from time to time to keep chicken and vegetables submerged. Strain through a collander lined with a double layer of cheesecloth. Discard all solids and cool the stock. Refrigerate overnight. Remove all fat from surface, reheat until fully liquid and pour into containers. The stock will keep up to 6 months in the freezer. Use for sauces and soups.

Tomato Coulis

(298 calories per cup)

A coulis is simply a reduced puree. This tomato version can be served hot or cold to complement many dishes and can be made smooth or chunky depending on its intended use. I have used it throughout the book as a base for pizza, lasagne, seafood, soups and chicken. When the season is at its peak and the market is bursting with fully ripe (and inexpensive), tomatoes make several batches of coulis and freeze in containers for later use. Makes 3 1/2 to 4 cups (nearly 1 litre).

1 teaspoon (5 mL) oil
1 large onion, finely chopped
1/3 cup (60 mL) shallots, finely chopped
4 cloves of garlic, finely chopped
16 ripe tomatoes (about 10 cups, 2.5 litres chopped)
1 14-oz can (398 mL) whole tomatoes
3 tablespoons (45 mL) finely chopped parsley
1 1/2 tablespoons (22 mL) fresh basil, chopped
1 1/2 tablespoons (22 mL) fresh oregano
or 1/2 tablespoon (7 mL) dried oregano
1 cup (250 mL) dry white wine
1 cup (250 mL) tomato juice
Pepper to taste.

Peel, seed and coarsely chop the tomatoes. Heat oil in large pan and saute onion, shallots and garlic for a few minutes until just golden. Add the rest of the ingredients and simmer for about 25 minutes until slightly thickened. Cool, then puree. I like my coulis a bit chunky. For a smoother sauce, it can be pureed a second time. Divide into 1 cup (250 mL) and 2 cup (500 mL) containers and freeze.

Tomato coulis has many uses including the following:

Primavera Pasta

Toss steamed broccoli, green beans and zucchini with lightly sauteed purple onion, mushrooms and sun-dried tomatoes or red peppers and mix with tomato coulis. Serve over fettucine noodles mixed with a little more coulis and sprinkle with freshly grated Parmesan cheese. Zap in the microwave for a few seconds to heat through.

Tomato Scallops

Poach scallops in a little clam juice, lemon and Pernod (optional) just until opaque. Keep hot. Heat some tomato coulis. Place 3 tablespoons (45 mL) of coulis on individual scallop shells and top with 4 or 5 scallops. Sprinkle with parsley and serve with a lemon wedge. Serve alone as an appetizer course, or with saffron rice, sauteed pea pods, mushrooms and shallots as a main course.

Comfort Food

Whenever we plan to entertain or for everyday family dining we turn most often to those recipes we feel comfortable with, recipes that have become our own classics. They may have been handed down from our grandmothers, those that friends have given you over the years, that you have tried and adapted from a magazine or that you have created on your own. All of the following favourites have one thing in common: they are low in fat and in total calories but they are nevertheless delectable and reliable — and bring compliments.

Shrimp and Scallop Seviche

(91 calories per serving)

A classic Mexican salad or appetizer served on a bed of butter lettuce. It can be prepared several hours in advance and it's rich, so small portions are advised. The combination of shrimp and scallops is particularly tasty. This also makes a delicious summer luncheon. Serves 4.

10 scallops (about 1/4 lb, 125 g), cut into small cubes
Juice of 3 limes
Juice of 1 lemon
2 teaspoons (10 mL) each of fresh green and red peppers, diced or 1 teaspoon (5 mL) each of dried red and green peppers
4 tablespoons (60 mL) chopped tomato
1 small garlic clove, pressed
3 tablespoons (45 mL) green onions, chopped
1 tablespoon (15 mL) ground coriander
1/4 lb (125 g) fresh baby shrimp

In a glass bowl combine scallops with lime and lemon juice. Marinate about 4 to 5 hours in the refrigerator until scallops are opaque. Add the rest of the ingredients and leave for an additional hour or so. Serve on bed of butter lettuce with wedges of lemon and lime.

Red Pepper Yogurt Mousse

(94 calories per serving)

Guests will never know that this yummy appetizer isn't loaded with butter, cream or cheese. It's simple to make and the slightly tart yogurt is enhanced by the sweet fresh red pepper and green onions.

Serves 8 to 10.

2 cups (500 mL) low fat yogurt, strained
1/4 teaspoon (1 mL) Dijon mustard
1/2 to 3/4 cup (125 to 180 mL) chopped green onion
2 medium red peppers
wholewheat Melba Toast

On the day ahead, strain yogurt in a cheesecloth-lined strainer overnight to remove excess liquid. Fold in mustard. Line a 2-cup (500 mL) mould or pan with plastic wrap, leaving extra draped over the edges. Pour half the yogurt mixture in, sprinkle with a layer of chopped roasted red peppers, leaving some for the top. Add a thin layer of green onion. Spread remaining yogurt on top, fold plastic wrap over and refrigerate. Just before serving, cover half the top with reserved red pepper, the other half with remaining green onions. Serve with Melba Toast.

To prepare peppers

Broil peppers about 6 inches (15 cm) from the heat source, turning frequently until they are black all over, about 8 to 10 minutes. Remove from grill and place in brown paper bag. Leave for several minutes, then remove and peel, cut open and remove seeds and ribs. Chop finely.

Broiled peppers can also be cut into strips and served with grilled fish or chicken. For extra colour, combine red, yellow and green peppers.

Marcelle's Pesto Mousse

(129 calories per serving as appetizer)
(323 calories per serving as lunch entree)

It's as light as a feather and smooth as velvet. Make it the day ahead, reheat and serve on wholewheat or water crackers. Our friends the McLeans served it as a quiche with a "crust" made from thinly-sliced zucchini.

Serves 10 as appetizer, 4 for main entree.

1/2 cup (125 mL) finely chopped green onion
1/4 cup (60 mL) finely chopped shallots (or substitute more green onion)
3 whole eggs
2 egg whites
2 cups (500 mL) low-fat ricotta cheese
Pinch Dijon mustard
Pinch fresh pepper
Pinch fresh nutmeg

Combine ingredients in a food processor and beat until smooth.

Pesto Topping

1 1/2 cups (375 mL) fresh basil leaves
1 large clove garlic, finely chopped
2 tablespoons (30 mL) toasted pine nuts
1 1/2 tablespoons (22 mL) freshly grated Parmesan or Romano cheese
1 tablespoon (15 mL) vegetable oil
Good pinch of pepper

Combine everything in food processor and set aside. (This basic pesto sauce can be used for pasta. It makes enough for 3/4 lb, 375 grams fettucine).

To prepare Mousse: Pour the ricotta filling into a 9 inch quiche pan sprayed with vegetable oil and bake at 375 degrees F (190 degrees C) for about 30 minutes or until firm on top. Remove from oven and spread pesto sauce evenly on top. Return to oven and bake for a few minutes longer to heat the topping. At this stage, the dish can be refrigerated and held for a day. Reheat at 350 degrees F (180 degrees C) for about 20 to 25 minutes. Guests spread the warm mousse on crackers for munching.

To make as a quiche, line lightly oiled pan with thin slices of zucchini before pouring in the filling and cut into slices to serve.

Hummus Spread

(12 calories per tablespoon)

This makes an excellent appetizer with warm pita bread and it's also good as a spread for pita-pocket sandwiches. The beans are an excellent source of protein. Makes about 2 cups (500 mL).

1/4 cup (60 mL) chopped green onion
1 clove garlic, pressed
1/2 teaspoon (2 mL) basil
1/2 teaspoon (2 mL) oregano
1/8 teaspoon (.5 mL) cumin
Pepper to taste
1 19-oz (540 mL) can garbanzo beans, drained and rinsed
2 tablespoons (30 mL) lemon juice
1/4 cup (60 mL) toasted sesame seed
2 tablespoons (30 mL) tahini paste

Saute onions, garlic herbs and spices in a little safflower oil. Add to rest of ingredients and blend quickly in blender or food processor. It should not be too smooth. Chill and serve. This will keep for days in the refrigerator.

Light Mayonnaise

(15 calories per teaspoon)

This light low-calorie version of mayonnaise serves as a base for sauces, dips and dressings. Fresh herbs and Dijon mustard enhance the taste. Makes about 1 cup (250 mL)

1/2 cup (125 mL) low fat yogurt, strained
1/2 cup (125 mL) low fat ricotta cheese, strained
1 tablespoon (15 mL) lemon juice
1/2 teaspoon (2 mL) Dijon mustard
Dash of Worcestershire sauce
Pepper to taste

Combine all in bowl and cream well with wire whisk. Store in refrigerator for up to a week.

Yogurt Salad Dressing

(19 calories per tablespoon)

A tangy dressing for spinach or assorted greens, tossed with a few toasted sesame seeds, grapefruit and orange sections and chopped green onions. The dressing will keep in the refrigerator for 3 to 4 days. The rice wine vinegar gives it a light taste.

1 cup (250 mL) low fat yogurt, strained overnight
1 teaspoon (5 mL) Dijon mustard
1 tablespoon (15 mL) oil
3 tablespoons (45 mL) green onions
3 tablespoons (45 mL) chopped parsley
2 tablespoons (30 mL) rice wine vinegar
Pepper to taste
A few drops of Worcestershire sauce
1 clove garlic, pressed
1/8 teaspoon (.5 mL) Hungarian sweet paprika
2 teaspoons (10 mL) dried dill
or 6 teaspoons (30 mL) fresh dill, chopped

Combine everything, mix well and store in refrigerator.

Stuffed Tomatoes

(143 calories per serving)

Greek in inspiration, these goes well with grilled chicken and seafood. Add a soup and a salad and they make a complete light luncheon. Served cold, they make an interesting appetizer course. Serves 6 to 8.

6 to 8 medium-size firm tomatoes
1 large onion, chopped
1 cup (250 mL) long grain brown rice
2 tablespoons (30 mL) raisins
2 tablespoons (30 mL) pine nuts
2 teaspoons (10 mL) dried marjoram
6 leaves fresh mint, chopped
or 1/2 teaspoon (2 mL) dried mint
2 tablespoons (30 mL) chopped parsley
2 cups (500 mL) chicken stock
Pepper to taste

With a sharp knife, carefully hollow out the tomatoes, being careful not to pierce the shells. Chop pulp. Saute onions in a little oil until soft. Add tomato pulp, rice, raisins and nuts and saute for a few minutes longer. Add herbs and chicken stock and bring to a boil, stirring well. Cover pan and simmer for about 30 minutes or until rice is tender and liquid almost all absorbed.

Pack mixture loosely into the tomato shells and place into a shallow baking dish along with about 1/2 inch (1 cm) of water. (Any extra stuffing can be cooked in a small casserole alongside, or refrigerated for later use.) Bake at 350 degrees F (180 degrees C) for about 20 minutes, just until tomato shells are tender. Don't overcook or the tomatoes will collapse.

Family Potluck Chicken

(401 calories per serving)

Whenever your refrigerator becomes full of little bits of leftover vegetables, try this roast chicken meal-in-one. Substitute whatever vegetables you have on hand for those specified here. Serves 8.

3 to 3 1/2 lb (1.5 to 2 kilo) roasting chicken
1 cup (250 mL) tomato coulis (see Index)
or 1 cup (250 mL) low-sodium tomato sauce
3 to 4 tablespoons (45 to 60 mL) tomato paste
1 1/2 cups (375) dry red or white wine
or 1 1/2 cups (375 mL) V-8 or tomato juice
2 cloves garlic, crushed
Pepper to taste
2 shallots, finely chopped
1/2 purple or white onion, sliced
Fresh or dry herbs to taste
such as basil, oregano, marjoram
3 tablespoons (45 mL) chopped parsley
4 sticks of celery, sliced thickly on diagonal
3 carrots, sliced 1/4 inch (6 mm) thick
1 cup (250 mL) fresh mushrooms, thickly sliced
1 or 2 zucchini, sliced 1/4 inch (6 mm) thick
1 or 2 pattypan or crookneck squash, sliced 1/4 inch (6mm) thick
1/2 small eggplant, unpeeled, in large cubes
2 to 3 tablespoons (30 to 45 mL) sun-dried tomatoes, thinly sliced
1/2 cup (125 mL) cherry tomatoes
1/2 cup (125 mL) canned artichoke hearts

As you can see, when it comes to vegetables, anything goes. Add broccoli, cauliflower, turnip, potatoes — just whatever you have. Put all the vegetables into a large Dutch oven. Clean chicken thoroughly, removing skin and all visible fat and place it, breast-side down, on top of the vegetables. Spoon some of the vegetables and liquid on top. Cover and bake at 350 degrees F (180 degrees C) for about 1 1/2 to 2 hours until chicken is tender. Remove chicken, slice and place on a large shallow serving dish, surrounded with the cooked vegetables. Serve with fettucine, baked potatoes, brown rice or couscous and the sauce from the vegetables.

Vegetable Curry

(204 calories per serving)

Simon Hoogewerf, Canadian champion 800 metre runner and Olympic competitor dons a chef's hat to prepare his mom's Dutch Indonesian recipe for a spicy curry dish that is a hit with all his athlete friends. Serves 6 to 8.

3 tablespoons (45 mL) safflower oil
2 onions, chopped
3 to 4 tablespoons (45 to 60 mL) curry powder or to taste
1 tablespoon (15 mL) curry paste (available at specialty counters)
1/4 cup (60 mL) brown sugar
Juice of 1 lemon
28-oz (796 mL) can of tomatoes, undrained
4 cups (1 litre) water
1 cup (250 mL) unsweetened medium-shred coconut
1 medium cauliflower
6 carrots
4 potatoes
1 cup (250 mL) peas
1/2 cup (125 mL) coriander seeds or to taste
1 tablespoon (15 mL) turmeric or to taste
1/4 cup (60 mL) unbleached flour
Pepper to taste
Optional: 1 cup (250 mL) of snow peas or broccoli tips

Saute onions in oil until soft but not brown. Add curry powder and paste and simmer for 10 minutes. While curry is simmering, chop vegetables and dust well with a mixture of flour and turmeric. Add vegetables to curry mixture and stir well. Add tomatoes, water, coconut, sugar and lemon juice. Bring to a boil, add coriander and pepper to taste. Simmer for ¾ hour. Add peas just before serving. This curry is better if made a day ahead. Reheat, adding peas at the last minute.

Serve with plain boiled rice, mango chutney, poppadums or chapatis and sour cream and side dishes of bananas, melon and nuts.

Cal-Mex Fiesta

(300 calories per serving)

This entertaining idea comes from Olympic runners Paul and Lynn Williams who acquired a taste for California-style Mexican cuisine while training in San Diego. Lynn, the Canadian record holder, won a bronze medal for the 3,000 metres at the Los Angeles Olympics; her husband Paul, also a Canadian record holder, is Canada's premier 5,000 and 10,000 metre runner. They both realize the importance of good nutrition and enjoy puttering in their kitchen to relax after training. Their fiesta makes a lively and informal evening with guests making their own fillings for stuffed tortillas.

Serves 6 to 8.

Fajitas

1 lb (500 g) chicken breast, deboned, skin removed and cut into 2-inch (5 cm) strips
1 lb (500 g) flank or rump steak, sliced across the grain in 2-inch (5 cm) strips
2 green peppers, thinly sliced
2 red peppers, thinly sliced
1 large onion, thinly sliced
1 green onion, chopped
1 clove garlic, chopped
1 strip ginger, peeled and chopped
12 large flour tortillas

Marinade

1/2 onion, chopped
1 clove garlic, smashed
1 teaspoon (5 mL) peeled, diced fresh ginger
1/4 cup (60 mL) water
1 1/2 teaspoons (7 mL) brown sugar
1 1/2 cups (375 mL) soy sauce
1/2 cup (125 mL) water

To make marinade: Place first four ingredients in blender and blend well. Add rest of ingredients. Pour over meat strips and leave to marinate for an hour or more.

Heat 2 tablespoons (30 mL) oil in skillet or wok. Saute green onions, garlic and ginger. Remove. Drain meats well, reserving liquid. Stir fry chicken until barely done; remove. Stir fry beef until barely done; remove. Place meats in separate skillets and cover with equal amounts of green and red peppers and onions. Pour 1/4 cup (60 mL) of marinade over each and sprinkle with 1 tablespoon (15 mL) oil.

Just before serving, place skillets under broiler and broil until sizzling. Serve still sizzling at the table. Guests use the meats and vegetables to stuff their own tortillas. (Serve tortillas warm: wrap them in a damp kitchen towel and place in warm oven for about half an hour). Serve with Mexican condiments, including salsa, green onions, shredded low-fat cheese such as Mozzarella, chopped tomatoes etc. To round out the meal, add Mexican Rice or Refried Beans, a fruit salad and sangria. Ole!

Williams' Mexican Rice

(136 calories per serving)

This dish can be made the day ahead and reheated. Serves 6 to 8.

2 tablespoons (30 mL) olive oil
1 cup (250 mL) chopped onion
2 cups (500 mL) uncooked white rice
2 cloves garlic, minced
1 cup (250 mL) chopped green pepper
1 cup (250 mL) chopped tomatoes
1 canned chili pepper, minced
or 1/4 teaspoon (1 mL) ground chili peppers
2 teaspoons (10 mL) chili powder
3 1/2 cups (875 mL) boiling water

Heat oil in large casserole and saute onions until soft. Stir in rice and garlic and cook until rice turns transparent. Add the rest of the ingredients. Cover and cook over low heat until rice is tender, about 25 minutes.

Lemon Brown Rice and Zucchini Pilaf

(120 calories per serving)

This is truly nutritious with a crunchy nut-like flavour enhanced by dill and lemon. It can be made the day ahead and reheated. Serves 6 to 8.

3 cups (750 mL) home-made chicken stock (see Index)
$1^1/_3$ cups (330 mL) long grain brown rice
Juice and zest of 1 lemon
$^1/_4$ cup (60 mL) chopped fresh dill
or 1 teaspoon (5 mL) dried dillweed
1 medium-size zucchini, cut into julienne strips and patted dry
1 clove garlic, crushed

The day before serving, combine in a saucepan the stock, rice, lemon zest, juice and dill. Cover, bring to a boil and simmer for 45 to 50 minutes until all liquid has been absorbed. Meanwhile, in a non-stick pan, cook zucchini and garlic with a teaspoon (5 mL) of water until barely tender. Add to rice and steam for about 5 minutes. Turn into a baking dish and refrigerate, covered, until ready to heat.

Bake at 350 degrees F (180 degrees C) until heated through.

Rabbit Stew with Eggplant

(243 calories per serving)

A gutsy stew, great with new potatoes and fresh green beans. Rabbit meat is very low in fat. Serves 6 to 8.

2 fresh rabbits, ribs and back removed, cut into serving portions
1 teaspoon (5 mL) safflower oil
2 sticks celery, chopped
1 14-oz (398 mL) can plum tomatoes
1 garlic clove, crushed
1/2 cup (125 mL) Marsala or Madeira wine or sweet sherry
Chicken stock to cover
1 medium eggplant, cut into 1 1/2-inch (3 cm) cubes

Lightly saute rabbit pieces in the oil in a large Dutch oven. Add celery and garlic and saute for a few minutes. Add Marsala and cook for a few minutes. Discard half of the juice from the canned tomatoes and add them to the pot along with chicken stock or water to cover. Bring to a boil and simmer for 15 to 20 minutes. Add eggplant and continue to cook until rabbit is tender. Remove rabbit and eggplant to a casserole dish and thicken the sauce by reduction (or add 1 tablespoon (15 mL) of cornstarch mixed with a little cold chicken stock). Pour sauce over rabbit. At this stage the dish can be covered and refrigerated. Reheat in a medium oven until bubbly hot.

Family Vegetable Soup

(240 calories per serving)

A meal in itself, along with a green salad, this is my family's favourite hearty soup. It's chock full of healthy vegetables and pasta or barley, all the nutrients necessary for energy plus! It's best made a day ahead of serving and freezes well. Serves 6 as basic meal.

1 teaspoon (5 mL) oil
1 medium onion, chopped
2 leeks, white parts only, chopped
2 cloves garlic, finely chopped
1 tablespoon each (15 mL) of fresh basil, marjoram and oregano
or 1 teaspoon (5 mL) each of dried herbs
1 cup (250 mL) pinto or red kidney beans
1 cup (250 mL) green beans, sliced on diagonal
2 carrots, cut on diagonal
2 stalks of celery, cut on diagonal
1 medium fennel bulb, sliced (optional)
1 medium zucchini, sliced 1/4 inch (6 mm) thick
6 cups (1.5 litres) chicken stock
or 6 vegetable cubes dissolved in 6 cups (1.5 litres) water
28-oz can (796 mL) tomatoes, chopped, juice included
1 cup (250 mL) tomato coulis, optional (see Index)
6 tablespoons (90 mL) pearl barley
or 1 cup (250 mL) small tube pasta

Soak beans overnight or bring to boil with enough water to cover and simmer for about 1 to 1 1/2 hours until beans are tender. Drain (Alternatively, use canned red kidney beans.) In a large Dutch oven, saute onion, leeks, garlic and herbs in the oil. Add all the rest of the ingredients except pearl barley or pasta and simmer, uncovered, for 1 hour. Add the beans, pearl barley or pasta and simmer for an additional hour if you're using barley, or 20 minutes if you're using pasta. Adjust seasonings, cool, then refrigerate or freeze. Reheat to serve. Vary the vegetables according to availability.

Red Snapper with Peppers

(185 calories per serving)

Don and Marcelle's red snapper entree always receives compliments when they serve it to friends. It can be prepared ahead of time and needs only a quick last minute steaming. Serve with Pommes Parisienne (see Index) and fresh asparagus. Serves 6 to 8.

2 lbs (1 kilo) thin (1/4 in.) red snapper fillets
2 teaspoons (10 mL) Spanish or Hungarian paprika
1/2 teaspoon (2 mL) each of chili powder, cumin and garlic powder
1/4 teaspoon (1 mL) black pepper
2 tablespoons (30 mL) vegetable oil
5 garlic cloves, peeled
2 green peppers, cut into strips
1 red pepper, cut into strips
1/2 cup (125 mL) chopped parsley
1/4 cup (60 mL) water

Blend all spices together, add oil and mix well. Roll snapper fillets in mixture and place on non-stick pan. Roll pepper strips in remaining mixture and arrange over snapper and sprinkle parsley on top. Add garlic cloves and water. Refrigerate until ready to serve. Simmer, covered, until liquid is evaporated and snapper is opaque. Don't overcook.

Vegetable Frittata

(405 calories per serving)

This robust vegetable pie can be served with or without the wholewheat crust. It can be made in advance but does not freeze well. It's perfect for using up leftovers. The wholewheat crust is ideal for fruit pies.

Serves 4 as a main meal, 8 as a first course.

Wholewheat Crust

1 1/4 cups (300 mL) wholewheat flour
2 tablespoons (30 mL) safflower oil
4 tablespoons (60 mL) low-fat cottage cheese, sieved
1 tablespoon (15 mL) toasted sesame seeds
Ice water

Mix all together, moistening with just enough ice water to form a ball. Roll out and line a 9-inch (23 cm) quiche pan, pinching the edges. Bake at 375 degrees F (190 degrees C) for 8 to 10 minutes.

Filling

3 eggs plus 2 egg whites, lightly beaten
1/2 cup (125 mL) low-fat yogurt, strained overnight in cheesecloth
2 tablespoons (30 mL) Parmesan cheese
Few dashes of Tabasco sauce
1/3 cup (80 mL) low fat cottage cheese, sieved
1/4 teaspoon (1 mL) Dijon mustard
1/4 cup (60 mL) fresh dill
or 1 tablespoon (15 mL) dried dill
3 tablespoons (45 mL) chopped parsley
1 tablespoon (15 mL) each of fresh basil and oregano
or 1 teaspoon (5 mL) each of dried herbs
Pepper to taste
2 tablespoons (30 mL) wholewheat flour
1/4 teaspoon (1 mL) baking soda

Blend all together and mix well.

Vegetables

1 teaspoon (5 mL) safflower oil
3 tablespoons (45 mL) chopped onion

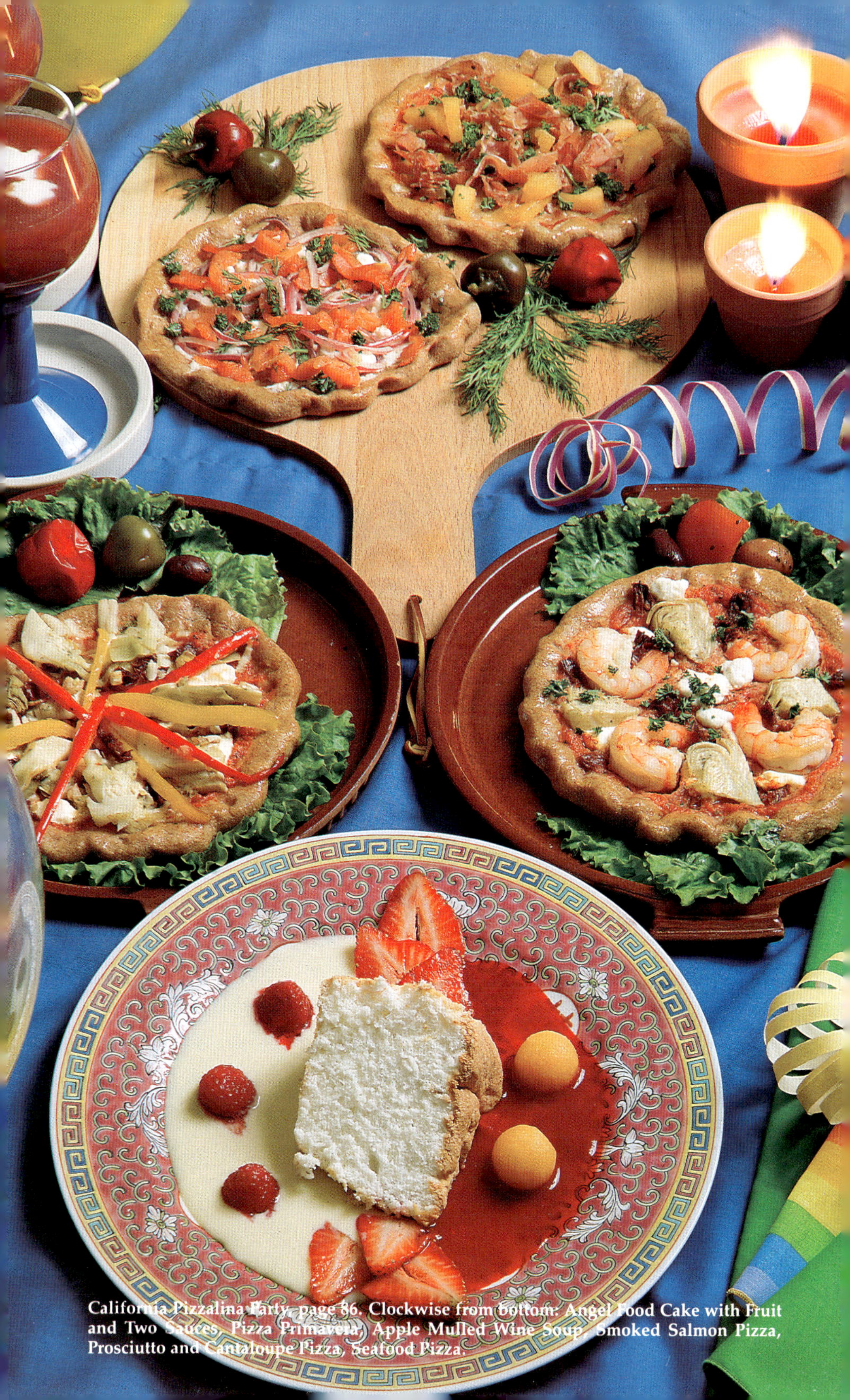

California Pizzalina Party, page 86. Clockwise from bottom: Angel Food Cake with Fruit and Two Sauces, Pizza Primavera, Apple Mulled Wine Soup, Smoked Salmon Pizza, Prosciutto and Cantaloupe Pizza, Seafood Pizza.

Fuel Foods, page 92. Clockwise from bottom: Salsa with Corn Chips, Graham Bread, Baked Stuffed Apples, Vegetable Basket with Yogurt Dip, Black Bean Soup.

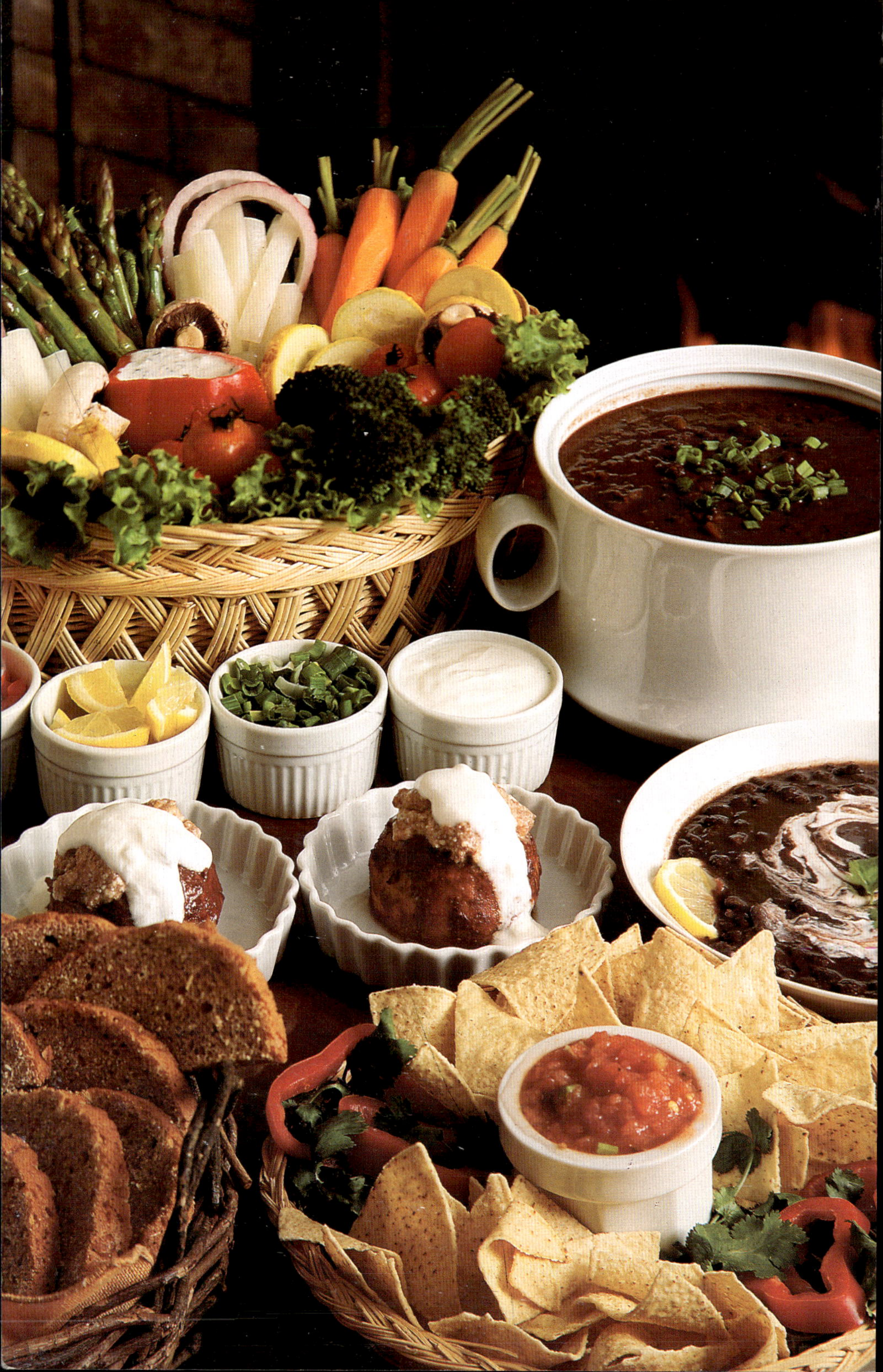

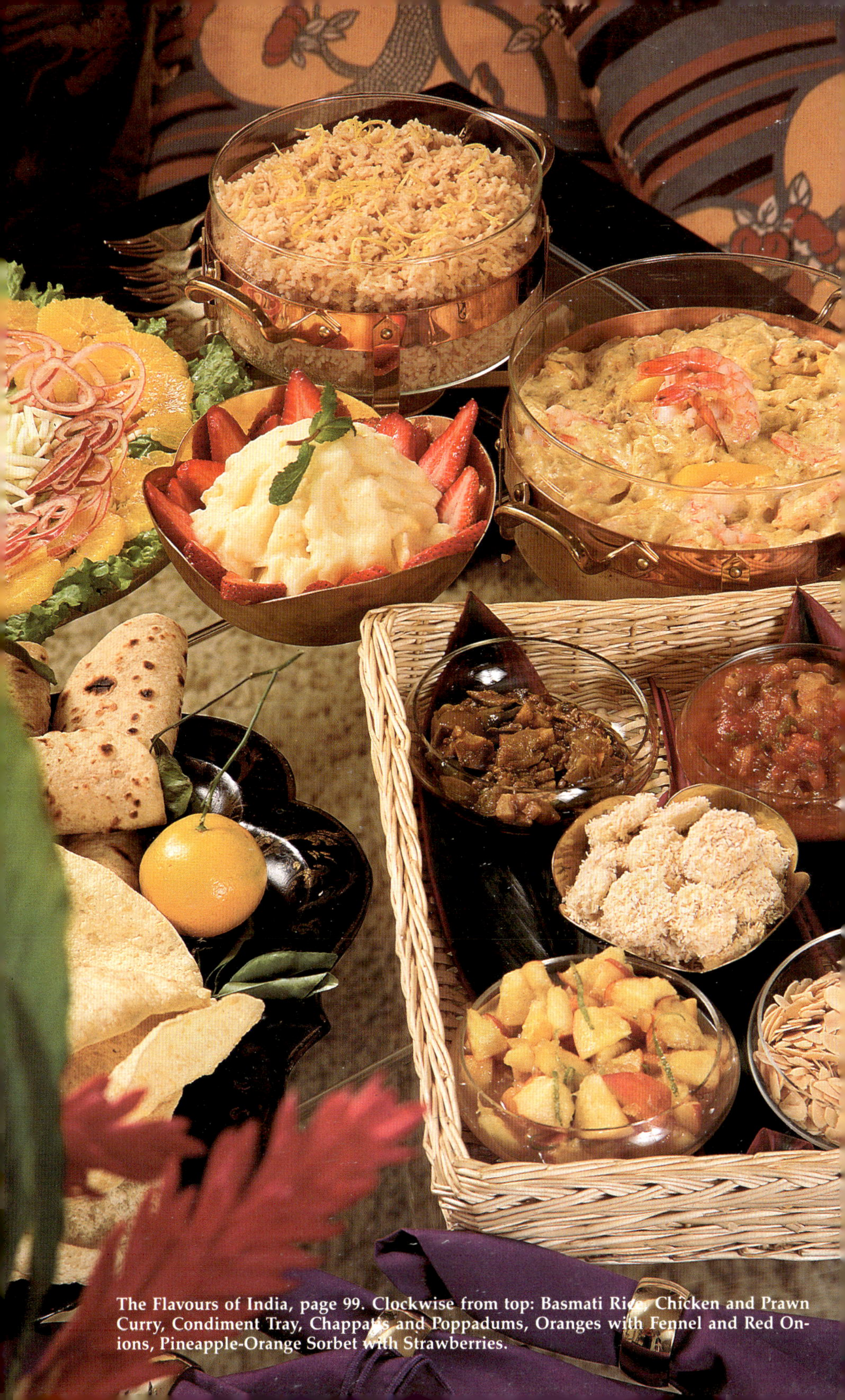

The Flavours of India, page 99. Clockwise from top: Basmati Rice, Chicken and Prawn Curry, Condiment Tray, Chappatis and Poppadums, Oranges with Fennel and Red Onions, Pineapple-Orange Sorbet with Strawberries.

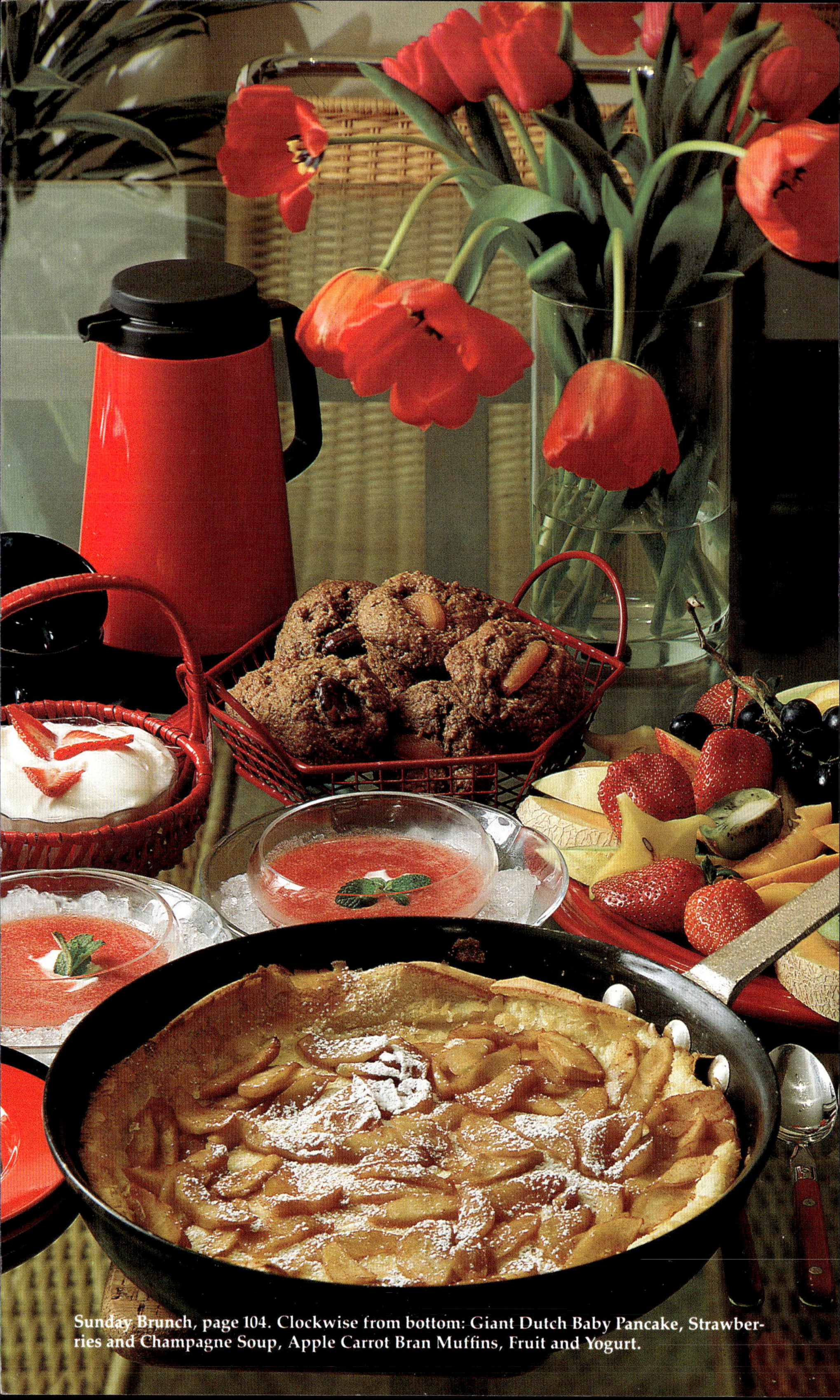

Sunday Brunch, page 104. Clockwise from bottom: Giant Dutch Baby Pancake, Strawberries and Champagne Soup, Apple Carrot Bran Muffins, Fruit and Yogurt.

1 tablespoon (15 mL) chopped shallots
1/2 green or red pepper, finely chopped
1/2 cup (125 mL) zucchini, sliced thinly
1 cup (250 mL) mushrooms, thinly sliced
3 cups (750 mL) fresh spinach, chopped
2 or 3 medium size, firm ripe tomatoes
sliced about 1/4 inch (6 mm) thick
1 tablespoon (15 mL) Parmesan cheese

Saute first five ingredients in the oil for a few minutes. Add spinach and mix just to blend and cook until spinach is limp. Set aside to cool. Fold into the filling and pour into the cooked crust, topping with a layer of tomatoes and sprinkling with cheese. Bake at 350 degrees F (180 degrees C) for about 40 minutes or until firm to touch.

Ratatouille

(46 calories per serving)

This dependable standby dish can be served hot or cold and goes well with chicken, grilled fish and rice. Serves 8.

1 teaspoon (5 mL) oil
1/2 cup (125 mL) chopped white or purple onions
2 cloves garlic, chopped
1 medium eggplant, unpeeled, cubed
1 to 2 tablespoons (15 to 30 mL) tomato juice
1 large zucchini, sliced 1/4 inch (6 mm) thick
1 cup (250 mL) sliced mushrooms
3 tablespoons (45 mL) each of fresh basil and oregano
or 1 tablespoon (15 mL) each of dried herbs
Pepper to taste
3 to 4 large tomatoes, peeled, seeded and cubed

Heat oil in large skillet and saute onions and garlic briefly. Add eggplant and cook for about 15 minutes, uncovered, stirring from time to time. Cover for a few minutes if it starts to dry out, adding a little tomato juice. Add zucchini, mushrooms, and herbs and cook for a few minutes, then add tomatoes. Cover and simmer for about 25 minutes. Cool, then keep in the refrigerator for 2 to 3 days. Serve hot or cold. It freezes well.

Middle Eastern Chicken

(269 calories per serving)

The aromatic spices used in Middle Eastern cuisine give this dish its exotic taste. Serve it with basmati or brown rice and some steamed vegetables or ratatouille. Serves 8.

4 to 5 lbs (2 to 2.5 kilos) chicken pieces, skin removed
1 tablespoon (15 mL) each of dried thyme, rosemary
1/4 teaspoon (1 mL) Dijon mustard
*1/4 teaspoon (1 mL) whole-seed French mustard**
3 cloves garlic, chopped
1 cup (250 mL) chopped onion
1 chopped shallot
1 teaspoon (5 mL) turmeric
1/2 teaspoon (2 mL) ground ginger
1/2 teaspoon (2 mL) cinnamon
1/2 teaspoon (2 mL) ground cloves
3 cups (750 mL) low-fat yogurt, strained overnight
Juice and zest of 1 lemon

Mix herbs and roll chicken pieces in them to coat. Combine the rest of the ingredients in a large shallow dish and put in the chicken pieces, coating each piece well. Cover and leave to marinate in the refrigerator overnight.

When ready to bake, remove chicken, leaving some of the marinade on each piece and place in casserole dish. Cover and bake at 350 degrees F (180 degrees C) for 30 minutes, basting frequently with reserved marinade. Uncover and continue baking until chicken is cooked, about 25 more minutes. Baste from time to time.

* This specialty mustard is made from white wine and whole mustard seeds and spices. It has a coarse texture and a distinctive taste — great for sauces and salad dressings.

Yogurt Coffeecake

(251 calories per serving)

Cooking confederate and friend Barb Watt, who has always loved my sour-cream coffeecake, came up with this low-fat adaptation. It's still yummy and freezes well. Serves 8 to 10.

1/3 cup (80 mL) corn oil margarine
3/4 cup (180 mL) fructose
1 whole egg and 2 egg whites
2 cups (500 mL) unbleached flour
1 teaspoon (5 mL) baking powder
1 teaspoon (5 mL) baking soda
1 cup (250 mL) low-fat yogurt
1/4 cup (60 mL) skim milk
1 teaspoon (5 mL) vanilla
2 teaspoons (10 mL) cinnamon
1 teaspoon (5 mL) nutmeg
1/4 cup (60 mL) brown sugar
1/2 cup (125 mL) raisins
1/2 cup (125 mL) chopped walnuts

Spray a 9 inch (2.7 litre) bundt pan with oil. Cream margarine and sugar until light, blend in eggs and vanilla and beat well. Sift together flour, baking powder and baking soda and fold into the creamed mixture along with the yogurt, working just until blended. Pour half the batter into the prepared pan. Mix together the spices, nuts, raisins and brown sugar and sprinkle half over the batter. Cover with remaining batter and sprinkle with remaining topping. Bake for 45 to 50 minutes at 350 degrees F (180 degrees C). Cool on wire rack, then invert onto plate. Serve warm.

Apple Brown Bread Pudding

(293 calories per serving)

Old-fashioned desserts from the pioneer days are experiencing a revival, in particular bread and rice puddings. Both are nutritious: high in calcium, low in fat. Serves 6.

1 tablespoon (15 mL) butter or margarine
3 large green apples, peeled, cored, grated
1/2 cup (125 mL) raisins
1 tablespoon (15 mL) lemon juice
1 teaspoon (5 mL) cinnamon
6 slices wholewheat bread
2 cups (500 mL) skim milk
1/2 cup (125 mL) brown sugar
1 egg, beaten
1 teaspoon (5 mL) vanilla

Melt butter in large frypan, add lemon juice and saute apples and raisins until apples are barely tender. Sprinkle with cinnamon. Cut bread slices into quarters. Spray a baking dish with non-stick coating and arrange bread and apple mixture in layers, sprinkling bread layers with the brown sugar. Beat egg with milk and vanilla and pour over. Bake at 350 degrees F (180 degrees C) until set and nicely browned on top, about 30 to 40 minutes. Serve with a dab of Creme Anglaise (see Index) or vanilla-flavoured yogurt.

Spanish Rice Pudding

(280 calories per serving)

Growing up in the Maritimes, I remember looking forward to a dish of warm and satisfying rice pudding as I walked home from school during the cold winter months. Serves 6.

4 cups (1 litre) skim milk
1 cinnamon stick
zest of $^1/_2$ orange (in strip)
1 cup (250 mL) short-grain rice
2 cups (500 mL) water
$^2/_3$ cup (160 mL) sugar
$^1/_4$ teaspoon (1 mL) vanilla
Cinnamon

Slowly bring milk to a boil with cinnamon stick and orange strip. Meantime, mix rice with the water and boil together for five minutes. Drain well. Reduce milk to a simmer, add rice and cook, partly covered (leave lid askew) for 15 minutes. Add sugar, stir well and continue to cook for 30 minutes or longer until rice is soft and liquid absorbed. It should be creamy. Stir in vanilla. Remove cinnamon stick. Turn into glass serving dish (or individual dishes) and sprinkle top with cinnamon. (For a decorative effect, shake it through a stencil). Serve warm, removing orange strip just before serving.

Strawberry Banana Freeze

(92 calories per serving)

Very similar to the Banana Revitalizer but with the additional goodness of strawberries.
Serves 4.

2 medium size ripe bananas
Juice of 1/2 lemon
1 cup (250 mL) frozen unsweetened strawberries
1/2 cup fresh orange juice
1 tablespoon (15 mL) fresh lemon juice
1 tablespoon (15 mL) creme de cassis (blackcurrant liqueur)

Peel bananas, dip in lemon juice and freeze until solid. Minutes before serving, slice frozen bananas and strawberries. Put bananas and fruit juices into the blender and whirl until smooth. Slowly add frozen strawberries, a few at a time, then blend in the creme de cassis. Serve immediately.

Art Phillips' Porridge-on-the-Run

(166 calories per serving)

Art Phillips and Carole Taylor lead active lives but take time to keep fit and healthy. Art believes the best way to guarantee a high energy day is to start with porridge. He cooks it in the microwave oven. It's quick and there is no pot to clean.
Serves one.

1/4 cup (60 mL) rolled oats
3/4 cup (180 mL) skim milk
Good pinch cinnamon
Pinch salt (optional)

Place ingredients in a deep cereal bowl and mix together. Microwave on high for about 2 1/2 minutes. Stir and let sit until it thickens a bit, about another 30 seconds. Top with sliced bananas or berries in season, or, for a power breakfast, a little granola. Serve with skim milk. (Avoid cream and brown sugar — you won't miss them after a while.)

For more servings, prepare extra bowls and allow a slightly longer cooking time.

CHAPTER 4

The New Diet in Depth

Carbohydrates

Goal: To increase carbohydrate intake from the present 46% to 58% of daily diet. The major change within this goal is to reduce intake of refined sugars from 18% to 10% and to increase complex carbohydrates from 22% to 42%. Simple or natural sugar intake should remain at 6%.

Carbohydrates are, chemically speaking, carbon, hydrogen and oxygen arranged in various combinations. There are two carbohydrate types: simple (sugars) and complex (starch). Simple carbohydrates are made of one or two sugar molecules and include sucrose, glucose, fructose and lactose. Table sugar is the disaccharide sucrose which accounts for about 70% of all sugar consumption. Most North Americans today consume about 600 calories of sugar a day, which equates to 128 pounds of sugar per person per year, a long way from the new goal of 40 pounds per year.

Complex carbohydrates are mostly starches, nature's energy stored largely in the form of seeds and roots. Starchy foods are generally thought of as high in calories, low in nutrients and therefore to be avoided in a weight maintenance or weight loss program. But in reality, carbohydrates contain no more calories per gram than proteins and only half as many as fat. Because they have a high content of both fibre and water, they can be of immense benefit to a weight maintenance program in that they supply bulk to appease the appetite.

To increase consumption of complex carbohydrates, we must increase the use of whole grains, rice, corn, dried peas and beans, couscous and buckwheat.

Perhaps today's favourite form of complex carbohydrates is pasta. This is made from hard spring wheat or durum refined to produce semolina. It contains 13% protein. Dried peas and beans contain almost no fat and are also high in protein as well as complex carbohydrate.

Fresh fruits and vegetables are obvious mainstays in the complex carbohydrate list. High in fibre and water content they add bulk which satisfies the appetite. Fresh or frozen fruits and vegetables are best; canning and cooking leach out many of the nutrients.

Fibre

Goal: To increase fibre intake to 25 to 30 grams daily.

As we increase the amount of complex carbohydrates in our diet, we will automatically increase the amount of fibre. Some studies indicate that a high fibre diet may reduce the incidence of cancer of the colon and rectum. While this claim is still unproven, there is no doubt of the benefits of fibre in terms of reducing constipation and hemorrhoids.

There are several types of fibre: cellulose, hemi-cellulose, pectin, lignin and gum. Fibres are undigestible, though about half are broken down in the intestines by natural bacterial fermentation and this can lead to a socially embarrassing side-effect of a high fibre diet: flatulence and gas in the bowel. This is marked in individuals who are in the process of changing their diet and may lessen in time. Pectin, found in many fruits and vegetables, plus the fibre in dried beans and oatmeal, appear to stimulate excretion of cholesterol, thus lowering its level in the bloodstream.

The recommended daily intake of 25 to 30 grams of fibre is easily achieved. For instance, an average serving of navy or garbanzo beans contains 8 grams; three-bean salad, a split-pea or lentil soup about 5 grams; vegetable soup, bran or corn muffins about 3 grams; wholewheat rolls, zucchini, corn, broccoli, carrots, cabbage or cauliflower, 2 grams per serving and celery, many fruits and tomatoes one gram per serving. Cucumbers, lettuce, white bread and pasta contain very little fibre, 0.5 grams per serving.

Sugar

Goal: To decrease the amount of refined sugars in our diet from 18% to 10%.

Simple sugars are to be avoided because of their high concentration of calories. For instance, one pound of apples weighs in at 263 calories; one pound of caramels at close to 1800 calories. A two-ounce chocolate bar has the same number of calories as three bananas. However, two thirds of the current intake of 600 calories of sugar per day comes from sugar hidden in other foods: one tablespoon of tomato ketchup contains one teaspoon of sugar; 12 ounces of cola contains 6 teaspoons of sugar, to give just two examples.

Honey, while not a processed sugar, contains fructose and glucose and is still a simple sugar source and should be accounted for as such. Molasses, the residue of the sugar refinement process, is an improvement over sucrose in that it contains calcium, iron and potassium but it still counts as a simple sugar. Fructose has gained interest in recent years because it is much sweeter than sucrose and thus less of it needs to be used for the same effect. A caloric saving of 30% can often be achieved. Fructose has another advantage in that is does not stimulate or require an insulin response in the diabetic.

Apart from obesity through high calorie intake, other hazards of excess simple sugar consumption are tooth decay, hypoglycemia, and maybe even heart disease. Excess sugars are converted to fat and this may contribute to arteriosclerosis.

We can reduce the amount of sugar in our diet by substituting fresh fruits or no-fat popcorn for sweet snacks and rich desserts. Cakes, pies and cookies should be avoided, along with all sugared soft drinks (substitute mineral water, diluted fruit juices or, in moderation, artificially sweetened soft drinks). Stop using sugar in coffee and tea. And inspect the labels of all prepared foods and cereals for high sugar content.

Protein

The new diet, you will remember, requires that protein consumption remain static at about 12% of daily intake. However, balancing the other categories in the diet will automatically change the source of this protein from animal to vegetable. Animal and dairy sources of protein tend to be very high in fat. The average 160-pound man requires only 57 grams of protein a day whereas normal North American consumption is around 100 grams. The 12% allowance is certainly a generous one. Vegetarians who eat no fish or meat should remember that proteins from individual vegetable sources are by themselves incomplete, i.e., they do not supply all the essential amino acids. For complete proteins the vegetable sources must be mixed, i.e., legumes and grain together, or legumes plus seeds.

Fat

Goal: To reduce fat consumption from 40% to 30% of total daily calorie intake.

Saturated, mono and polyunsaturated fats should each account for 10% of this total. Cholesterol intake should be limited to keep blood cholesterol levels below 200 mg per decilitre.

The American Cancer Society's recent interim report suggests that avoidance of obesity and reduction of total fat intake may lessen the risk of breast, colon and prostate cancers. Statistics from the period between 1956 and 1976 (when 50% of Americans altered their eating habits as well as increased their exercise and decreased smoking) show that for the first time in this century the death rate from heart disease and strokes decreased. The actual cause of this reduction is unclear but it does seem to be associated with changes in lifestyle and with the decreased intake of dietary fat.

Saturated fats are more troublesome than unsaturated. They come mostly from animal sources and are mainly solid at room temperature. Examples of these are butter, cheese, chocolate, egg yolk, meat, milk fat and hydrogenated vegetable shortening. Unsaturated fats come largely from vegetable sources and are liquid at room temperature. Examples of mono-unsaturated fats are olive oil, cashews and peanuts. Polyunsaturated fats include almonds, corn oil, fish oil, soft margarine, safflower oil, soybean oil and sunflower oil. Saturated fats increase the blood cholesterol level while polyunsaturated fats lower it and mono-unsaturated fats have a neutral effect.

Perhaps the most troublesome of the fats is cholesterol. Like all fats, cholesterol is not water soluble and is transported in the blood by a protein carrier. Once linked to the protein it is called a lipoprotein. Lipoproteins deliver fats to fat depots in the body and cholesterol to cells. There are several types of lipoprotein: high density or HDL which seems to protect individuals against coronary artery disease, low density or LDL and very low density, VLDL. The low density lipoproteins are responsible for clogging of the arteries or arteriosclerosis. Some 70% of cholesterol is low density.

A diet high in saturated fats will induce increased production of low density lipoproteins in the liver, while increased use of polyunsaturated fats favors production of beneficial high density lipoproteins. Obese people have low percentages of HDL, but it will increase as their weight decreases. Exercise such as jogging increases HDL levels.

Recently the increased use of polyunsaturated fats has come into question since some studies of both animals and humans suggest increased risk of cancer. However, Eskimos who eat large quantities of polyunsaturated fats have no increased cancer risks. In general, then, one does not wish to increase polyunsaturated fat intake but simply to reduce all fat. And given a choice, to use polyunsaturated fats over saturated.

Reduction of fat can be achieved in the following ways: first, by cutting down on the amount of red meats or using only lean cuts such as sirloin or pork tenderloin, and trimming all visible fat. Veal and poultry, particularly young poultry, are generally low in fat, as are most fish and shellfish. Sole is probably the least fatty: 90% of its calories come from protein, only 10%

from fat, compared to a well- trimmed T-bone steak at 50% fat and poultry, 31% fat. Limit portion sizes of meat, fish and poultry to 2 to 3 oz (60 to 90 g) per serving. Generally speaking, avoid bacon, ham, spare ribs, hamburger, duck, goose, frankfurter, luncheon meats and most forms of sausage. Avoid liver, heart, kidney, sardines, anchovies and fish roe, all of which are high in cholesterol. Broil or roast meats to allow the fat to drip off and when making a meat-based soup stock, chill the stock well then skim off all the fat.

A hidden source of fat is often found in the cooking process. Take the potato, for instance. Half a pound of baked potato without any dressing contains 120 calories; the same amount of potatoes as French fries contain 620 calories and as potato chips, 1200 calories.

When it comes to dairy products, use skim milk and buttermilk (only 2 of the 88 calories in an 8-ounce glass of skim milk come from fat, compared with 77 of the 159 calories in a similar glass of whole milk); skim or low-fat yogurt; fruit ices instead of ice cream (even sherbet contains 2% fat). Totally avoid whipping cream which has 38% fat and light cream, 20% fat. Cream cheese is 37% fat and sour cream 18% fat. Gouda, Double Gloucester, and Edam are all lower in fat content than Cheddar which is 30% fat. Goat cheese is only 20% fat and some Mozzarella only 15% fat. Low fat cottage cheese is your best bet here.

Avoid animal fats such as butter and lard. Substitute vegetable oils and margarines where the polyunsaturated to saturated ratio is greater than 2 to 1. Don't use hydrogenated polyunsaturated fats because the hydrogenating process makes them more saturated. Vegetable oils that are acceptable are safflower, walnut, sunflower and unhydrogenated corn oil. Use olive oil, a mono-unsaturated fat, sparingly and avoid the use of coconut and peanut oil totally. Commercially baked goods are most probably high in saturated fats as are commercial salad dressings. Chocolate, nuts, seeds, peanut butter and avocados should be severely restricted or avoided.

Reduce the number of eggs consumed to no more than 4 per week. One egg contains 250 mgs of cholesterol, almost the total daily quota of 300 mgs. Only the egg yolk contains cholesterol so for recipes that call for whole eggs, simply substitute twice the number of egg whites.

Fats in Fast Foods

North Americans today eat almost half their meals in restaurants and spend about $10 billion a year in fast food outlets. Can we eat healthily at a fast food restaurant? It's not easy. A hot dog has 135 calories of fat, a 6-inch square of pizza, 135 fat calories, one fried chicken thigh, 171 fat calories. A quarter pounder with cheese, french fries and a milk shake add up to 1130 calories (almost half your daily needs) with fat content a staggering 42 %. What about a fillet of fish burger instead of the beef? This leads (because of the deep frying) to an even higher fat percentage, a shocking 52%, even though total calories are reduced by 100. When people realize the benefits of a 58 — 30 — 12 diet (58% carbohydrate, 30% fat, 12% protein) the fast food outlets will have to change. The trend is there already. There are several successful chain establishments where the offerings are hearty soups, salads, breads and fresh fruits, and these, I predict, will continue to thrive.

Vitamins and Minerals

A well-balanced diet will generally suppy all the vitamins and minerals the body needs although there are a few which might be deficient, particularly in women. These are the B complex vitamins, iron and calcium. Most of the body's calcium is in the bones. It has long been noticed that women as they age frequently suffer from osteoporosis or thinning of the bones, a condition which leaves the bones brittle and susceptible to fracture. The causes of this, while not entirely clear, seem to be associated with decreased levels of exercise, with the aging process, with loss of the female hormone estrogen after menopause and calcium deficiency in the diet.

In 1973 a Nutrition Canada survey showed that women over 65 took in fewer than 600 mg of calcium a day instead of the recommended 1500 mg. (For the population at large, recommended daily dosage is between 1000 and 1200 mg.) Calcium is easily added to the diet: an 8-ounce glass of skim milk contain 300 mg of calcium. The addition of two cups of skim milk and 8 ounces of plain yogurt (275 mg) a day to their regular diet would ensure that these post-menopausal women receive ample calcium. Another way they can help prevent osteoporosis is through exercise such as walking or swimming which stimulates bone deposition. It should be noted that calcium absorption is inhibited by alcohol and caffeine. An excess intake of protein may increase the loss of calcium from the body.

Iron deficiency, particularly in young women, appears to be relatively common. Iron deficiency anemia is believed to be the commonest deficiency among North Americans, affecting some 5% of women, and is prevalent world wide. Sufferers are most likely to be vegetarians, blood donors, new mothers and those engaged in heavy exercise. Since the normal diet contains 6 mg of iron for every 1000 calories, and the daily caloric intake for women is between 1500 and 2000 calories, this leads to an iron intake between 9 and 12 mg, only 50% of the recommended levels.

Iron comes from two dietary sources, animal and vegetable. The foods richest in assimilable iron are red meats and organ meats, but these are reduced in the new diet because they contain high levels of fat. Iron from vegetable sources is difficult to absorb. Iron from grains and other carbohydrates is bound to the undigestible fibre and will be mostly excreted. Absorption will be helped by mixing vegetable sources of iron with animal iron and with food containing vitamin C. Good sources of vegetable iron include whole grain and enriched breads and cereals, dark green leafy vegetables and dried fruits, beans and peas. Tea interferes with optimal absorption of iron.

It is unwise for anyone to take supplemental iron without proper medical diagnosis because a small but significant number of people have a genetic disorder in which high levels of iron are stored in the body. Supplemental iron in this case could be dangerous, even lethal.

Salt

Goal: To decrease salt intake to 5 grams a day.

Salt intake has come under scrutiny lately because of its direct and proven association with hypertension (high blood pressure). For example, Eskimos who typically take in only 2 grams of salt a day show absolutely no signs of high blood pressure whereas in Japan, where salt intake is 28 grams a day, 40% of the population suffer from high blood pressure. Salt intake in North America currently equals 15 pounds per person per year or 15 grams (4 teaspoons) per day. The actual physiological need is 0.5 grams. The McGovern Committee recommendations are for 5 grams per day. There is never any need to add salt to food because there is enough salt present in food naturally. The only exceptions to this are for athletes or workers in extraordinarily hot climates who lose greater than three quarts of sweat per day, equivalent to 6 lbs of weight loss.

To achieve the goal of less than 5 grams of salt per day: use no salt on the table; decrease or eliminate salt in cooking; choose low-sodium processed foods and check all labels for high salt content. Don't use water softeners on tap water; avoid antacids which are high in sodium. Baking powder and baking soda are additional sources of salt in baked foods.

Water

Water is perhaps the most vital nutrient of all foods, a fact often neglected in discussions of diet. It represents some 65% to 75% of body weight in males. (Females have a higher percentage of body fat and 10% less water). Water is necessary to regulate the internal environment of our bodies, for heat regulation and for elimination. Daily intake and output of fluids should be equal. We should each drink between 6 to 8 8-ounce glasses of fluid per day.

About half of North Americans have access to fluoridated water, either natural or fortified. Fluoridation of water supply leads to a 66% reduction in tooth decay and a decreased incidence of osteoporosis and yet, despite conclusive medical evidence, the other half are deprived of this protection because of a strong antifluoridation movement.

World-wide concern about water pollution has led to increased use of bottled water. While Canadians do not yet have to be concerned about the purity of their water supply, in the U.S., bottled water represents a $30 million industry. About three quarters of the bottled water sold is not natural mineral water; it may be fortified mineral water, or simply fortified or treated tapwater. In some cases, mineral water can be very high in sodium. The best kinds of bottled water are likely natural spring water containing calcium, magnesium, potassium and sodium in varying amounts.

Club soda is tap water artificially carbonated. Seltzer water is thrice-filtered water with added carbonation, no salts, no preservatives, no sugars, no flavourings. Soft drinks represent a major source of empty calories: an 8-oz serving of cola contains 6 teaspoons of sugar or 120 calories, the regular 12-oz bottle, 9 teaspoons of sugar and 180 calories. Increased consumption of soft drinks in North America has been phenomenal. In 1900, soft drinks averaged 10 8-oz servings per person per year. By 1978 this had risen to 577 servings, a $10 billion wholesale business, 63% of it from colas and only about 11% from diet soft drinks. Soft drinks account for the consumption of 23 pounds of sucrose per person per year or 14% of our annual sugar consumption. The caloric value of fruit juices is similar to that of soft drinks but they at least contain vitamins and minerals. Since the main requirement of our bodies is water, thirst may best be assuaged by plain water or small quantities of fruit juices, diluted perhaps in the ratio of 7 parts of water to one of juice.

Smoking

Dr. Thomas Pearson of Johns Hopkins Medical School predicts that the pratice of smoking will cease in North America by the year 2000 and one can easily see a marked change in public opinion and legislation that could well lead to this. Lung cancer was directly linked to cigarette smoking in the 1960s. It is thought that one third of all cancer in North America and Europe is related to the use of tobacco yet in spite of this, some 14% of all North American physicians continue to smoke, an indication of the tremendous addictive properties of nicotine. Children of smokers suffer a 65% increased risk of cancer and non-smoking adults living in the same household as a smoker have a 50% increased risk. Smoker's risk of death is seven times greater than that of a non-smoker. These risks come not only from lung cancer but from chronic lung diseases such as emphysema as well as diseases of the coronary arteries. The good news is that this increased risk of mortality decreases immediately once one gives up smoking. The decrease is only partial in each year after stopping smoking but after 15 years the risk has diminished almost to that of a non-smoker's.

Dr. James Middle, a consultant in medicine at Eastbourne District Hospital in England is trying to stop smoking by appealing to the smoker's vanity. He reports in the British Medical Journal that smoking causes ''smoker's face'', which is characterized by wrinkles, a leathery skin and an orange-purple complexion.

Alcohol

Alcohol is the major mood-altering drug used in North America. Only 9% of adults use tranquillizers regularly, 7% sleeping pills and 3% stimulants. Alcohol is a depressant which initially disinhibits the user by releasing emotional control. High intake of alcohol over a short time period can lead to coma or death. Heavy use of alcohol weakens the heart muscle and causes high blood pressure. It has a toxic effect on the brain, heart, liver and gastro-intestinal tract. Sustained use can lead to cirrhosis of the liver and ultimately to liver failure. Alcohol can aggravate existing peptic ulcers and also inhibit the absorption of essential nutrients from the diet, causing malnutrition and further aggravation of the liver. Sexual performance is reduced because alcohol inhibits production of the male sex hormone testosterone. And for the unborn child, it can cause heart malformation and mental retardation. On the other hand, the moderate use of alcohol, defined as one to two drinks per day, seems statistically to decrease the risk of coronary artery disease.

The effects of alcohol are responsible for more than half the motor vehicle accidents in North America and account for some 20,000 deaths per year and thus it is vital to be aware of the amount of alcohol needed for intoxication. One bottle of beer or $1^1/_2$ ounces of distilled spirits are considered one drink. One to two drinks per hour will lead to a blood alcohol reading of 0.01. This is not considered intoxicated and driving a car is probably safe. Three to four drinks per hour equals a reading of 0.05; this may be intoxication and caution should be shown in the decision to drive. Five to six drinks per hour gives a blood alcohol reading of 0.1; intoxication is highly likely and driving is not advised. Seven or more drinks per hour gives a reading of 0.15; intoxication is definite and driving is absolutely prohibited. Drivers apprehended by the police for drunken driving show average blood alcohol levels of 0.2.

In terms of nutrition, while one gram of fat is equal to 9 calories and one gram of carbohydrate and of protein to 4 calories, alcohol has 7 calories per gram. This means that 12 oz of regular beer has 150 calories, light beer 95, $3^1/_2$ oz wine 87, $1^1/_2$ oz of 80-proof rum 97. The mixer rings in 96 calories per 8 ounces. All alcohol is burned in the liver. It is not converted to fat, though beer and wines also contain unfermented carbohydrates which add calories.

The typical hangover from excess alcohol use is caused by the direct toxic effect of alcohol on the brain, along with dehydration, swollen cranial arteries which cause nausea, and vomiting from gastrointestinal irritation. Scotch whiskey, bourbon, red wine and brandy contain high levels of contaminants and other chemicals which contribute to the typical hangover headache. The best remedy for a hangover is to drink plenty of water and to rest. Social drinking will be more pleasurable (at least the next day) if you eat before drinking, avoid the use of salt which will stimulate thirst, add lots of mix and limit yourself to one drink per hour. In between drinks, ask for plain soda.

Caffeine

Caffeine is another important drug used by Canadians. It is very popular because it decreases fatigue by stimulating the central nervous system. More seriously, it increases the heart rate and rate of respiration, metabolism and heart stimulation. It also dilates the coronary arteries, increases muscle co-ordination and stimulates the kidney, acting as a powerful diuretic. Some 500,000 Canadians drink more than 7 cups of coffee a day. Regular use of 350 mg of caffeine a day, equal to 4 cups, will induce dependency in that withdrawal will cause headaches, drowsiness and lethargy and, after 12 to 16 hours of withdrawal, nervousness and depression. High doses of caffeine can cause delirium. However, there is so far no proof that high levels of caffeine alone produce heart disease or cancer. The role of caffeine in inducing cardiac arrhythmia (irregular heart beat) or peptic ulcers is uncertain, although it certainly seems to affect my heart.

Each 6-oz cup of brewed coffee contains 83 mg of caffeine; a cup of instant coffee has 60 mg while decaffeinated coffee has only 3 mg. Brewed leaf teas have between 41 and 81 mg of caffeine per serving; instant tea, 28 mg; 12 oz of cola has 72 mg caffeine, 6 oz of cocoa , 10 mg and 1 oz of chocolate, 5 to 10 mg.

It should be noted here that herbal teas, while not containing caffeine, are not innocuous. By definition, they contain herbs with specific medicinal aims. Some are cathartic, some allergenic, some stimulate the kidneys, some have a toxic effect on the central nervous system and some have poisonous qualities. Most herbal teas are intended for infrequent and medicinal use. They should not be used routinely as a beverage.

Milk is a common beverage and has a wholesome image. An 8-oz serving of whole milk contains 8 grams of protein, 8 grams of fat and 11 grams of carbohydrate for a total of 159 calories. It is fortified with vitamins A and D and contains about 120 mg of sodium. An 8-ounce glass of 2% milk represents 120 calories, skim milk (less than 0.5% fat) about 88 calories. Buttermilk has a low fat content. Yogurt can be made from whole, 2% or skim milk treated with a bacterial culture and has the added advantage of lowering the body's cholesterol level. Recent observations of Masai tribesmen in Kenya seem to indicate that milk and milk products such as yogurt consumed in quantities of two to four quarts a day limit cardio-vascular disease by lowering cholesterol levels. This effect has been confirmed in studies on both animals and humans but so far this "milk factor" has yet to be identified.

A Look at Lifestyle

Moderating the diet I know can make a tremendous difference to our levels of health and fitness. But diet is not everything. We should always keep in mind, for instance, that among younger men and women, motor vehicle accident is the major cause of death and that alcohol is implicated in over 50% of all motor accidents. Half of all spinal cord injuries are due to motor vehicle accident. The avoidance of alcohol, the practice of defensive driving and the use of seat belts are therefore urged.

Tranquillity is better than stress. There appears to be some truth to the theory that there may be a coronary-prone behaviour pattern known as the Type A personality. He or she is described as "struggling incessantly to achieve more and more in less and less time against the opposing efforts of others.'' These people have explosive behaviour, accelerated speech, a heightened pace of living, are impatient with illness, concentrate on more than one activity at once, are preoccupied with themselves, and have a strong tendency to compete, challenging others even in non-competitive situations. Individuals with these behaviour traits are often so deeply committed to their professions that other aspects of their lives are ignored.

On the other hand, the Type B personality is more relaxed, unhurried, mellow, satisfied and tends to flow with the stream of life instead of struggling against it. The risk of heart disease is 2.9 times greater in the Type A versus the Type B personality.

Probably none of us falls into pure Type A or pure Type B patterns and there is no question in my own mind that I have elements of both. Looking back, I can see that the times when my heart was acting up were also the times when I had been on the go and under pressure and committed to two or three deadlines at once, with no chance of easily achieving them. I also think I did (and perhaps still do) tend to challenge and compete with others. This kind of stress is self-created because I and others enjoy it; we look for it. It is purely a question of moderation, keeping these levels of excitement and challenge under control. Today, I like to think that I can be relaxed, unhurried and mellow. At least, I'm working on it.

In the early 1970s Belloc and Breslow described the Seven Health Practices:

1. Sleep, usually 7 to 8 hours.
2. Breakfast, eat almost always.
3. Snacking, seldom or never.
4. Weight, maintain a desirable weight, for men not more than 20% above ideal weight; for women, not more than 10% above ideal weight.
5. Exercise, on a frequent basis.
6. Alcohol, not more than 4 drinks a day.
7. Tobacco, never smoke cigarettes.

If a man of 55 has followed these seven rules all his life, then from a physiological point of view he will have a life expectancy of someone 20 years younger.

Exercise

This is the place I would like to talk about Rule Number 5, exercise frequently. I promise to touch the subject only lightly, not because it is unimportant but because this is principally a cookbook. Dr. Roy Shepherd of the University of Toronto has stated that a lifelong practice of regular physical activity can delay the onset of physiological aging by about 10 years. Guidelines established by the American College of Sports Medicine for the maintenance of cardio- vascular health call for exercise three to five times a week for durations of 20 to 40 minutes at 70% of maximum heart rate. This activity should be sustained, such as in walking, running, swimming and cycling so that the heart rate is maintained steadily throughout the exercise period. Other forms of exercise such as golf and tennis are also acceptable but may have to be done longer in order to obtain the cardio-vascular benefits.

To establish your exercise pulse rate, subtract your age from 220 and take 70% of the answer. In my case, age 53, the maximum heart rate is 167, and my exercise heart rate is 117 beats per minute. If I were to exercise at this heart rate for 30 to 40 minutes three to five times week, I would meet the basic requirement for cardio-vascular health. In fact, that's pretty well what I do. I choose to run, usually for 40 to 50 minutes, often at lunch time, twice or three times a week. I supplement this with some trunk and upper body exercises such as push-ups and sit-ups.

To start a cardio-vascular fitness program, first check with your family doctor. Walking would be a good choice of activity. Begin walking briskly three times a week, say on Tuesdays, Thursdays or Saturdays, allowing recovery days on Wednesdays, Fridays and Sundays, with Mondays as "days off". Start walking for 5 minutes and increase by 5 minutes each session until you are walking for 45 to 50 minutes or longer. Choose a park or scenic route for best enjoyment.

If you choose to run, set aside 45 minutes three times a week and imagine that each 45 minutes is divided into 9 five-minute sessions. In each session for the first week run for only 1/2 minute and walk the other 4 1/2 minutes. (Total running time = 4 1/2 minutes; walking = 40 1/2 minutes). Increase running times per session by 1/2 minute in each of the following weeks so that by week 5 you are running for a total of 22 1/2 minutes, walking for 22 1/2 minutes and by week 10, you are running for the whole 45 minutes. Remember that the running segments should be easy. You should be able to converse with a partner to "pass the talk test". Pulse rate should be 120 to 140 for most adults. Pushing too hard will defeat the purpose of cardiovascular training.

I find I enjoy running in the woods and parks. The softer, undulating paths suit me better than man-made asphalt or concrete roadways. Today's sturdy running shoes, however, make the latter possible, and in winter there is often no alternative. I supplement running with three basic strength drills: static V sit-ups, parallel squats and classic push-ups. None of these require special equipment. I do these exercises after my run two or three times a week.

Static V Sit-up

Lie down, face up, on a soft surface such as a carpet. Bend the knees to 90 degrees and the hips to 45 degrees. Do not hook or hold the feet down. With hands behind the head, press small of the back to the floor and roll head, neck and trunk up until trunk and thighs form a V profile. Hold this position for 20 seconds, then roll down. Rest momentarily and then repeat for a total of 6. This is tougher than it looks. I started off with 6 repeats of only 5 seconds' duration, and added a second each session. It took me five to six weeks to reach the target of 6 repeats of 20 seconds. At the beginning, I could not raise my trunk off the ground at all. But don't strain. Just get your head, neck and shoulders up first and your trunk will gradually come too. This exercise does wonders for the back since it strengthens abdominal muscles, the key to good posture.

Parallel or Half Squats

Start in a standing position, feet parallel and about shoulder width apart. Drop to a squat so the thigh is parallel to the floor. Keep heels on the floor, arms in front for balance. Start slowly, keeping your knee over your large toe (not over the inside of your foot) as you drop. Rise and repeat. I started with 3 sets of 5 repetitions and increased them by one until I reached my goal of 3 sets of 20. I take a small break after each set. This drill keeps the thigh muscles strong and is very helpful in avoiding knee problems.

Anyone who is just beginning a fitness program could start with a quarter squat, bending the knees only halfway to the parallel position. This could be done for several months before you try the half squat. Remember to start slowly.

Classic Push-up

There is nothing sacred about this or the other exercises we have described. There are many good programs involving weight machines and other resistance equipment but push-ups require nothing other than yourself and the floor. They are truly portable, travelling with you on business and vacation trips. I choose to do 40 push-ups, usually 2 sets of 20. I lie face down with my hands under my shoulders, weight on my toes and push up and down. I started with 2 sets of 5 push-ups and increased one per set until I reached my goal.

Hopefully this basic program of running and exercising three times a week will allow me to enjoy skiing, hiking and travel for many years to come.

Index to Recipes

A
Aileen's Oatmeal Hearts 28
All-Season Zucchini Dill Soup 30
Almonds, Toasted 102
Angel Food Cake 91
Angel Hair Pasta, with Crab, etc. 43
Antipasto 47
Apple Brown Bread Pudding 128
Apple Carrot Bran Muffins 107
Apple Mulled Wine Soup 87
Apple Sauce 106
Apples, Baked, Stuffed 97
Apricot Souffle, Hot 44
Art Phillips' Porridge-on-the-Run 130
Asparagus, Green Peppercorn Dressing 71

B
Baked Stuffed Apples 97
Banana Ice 22
Bananas in Toasted Coconut 102
Basmati Rice 102
Black Bean Soup 96
Blackberry Ice 81
Blue Cheese — Walnut Salad 58
Bread
  Graham 95
  Hearty Peasant 37
  Wholewheat Bagel Crisps 77
Bulgar Rice Pilaf 72

C
Cabbage Rolls, Stuffed 38
Cal-Mex Fiesta 118
Carob Crispies 98
Carrot and Yam Puree 66
Chicken
  Chicken and Prawn Curry 101
  Chicken Stock 108
  Family Potluck Chicken 116
  Lemon Grilled Chicken 70
  Middle Eastern Chicken 126
  Oriental Chicken Salad 21
Chocolate Souffle 60
Chocolight Cake 67
Chutney, Peach 102
Coffee, Spiced 34
Coffeecake, Yogurt 127
Cookies
  Carob Crispies 98
  Oatmeal Hearts 28
Coulis, Tomato 108
Couscous 33
Creme Anglaise 80
Cucumber-Yogurt Soup, Chilled 36
Curry Sauce 25
Curry, Vegetable 117

D
Desserts
  Apple Brown Bread Pudding 128
  Apples, Baked, Stuffed 98
  Banana Ice with Raspberry Puree 22
  Blackberry Ice 81
  Chocolate Souffle 60
  Chocolight Cake 67
  Dried Fruit Compote 34
  Hot Apricot Souffle 44
  Jennifer's Angel Food Cake 91
  Lemon Slush 50
  Melon and Raspberries in Galliano 85
  Oranges in Sangria 73
  Pineapple-Orange Sorbet 103
  Poached Pears 80
  Shimmering Strawberry Goblets 40
  Spanish Rice Pudding 129
  Srawberry-Banana Freeze 130
  Tropical Mousse 56
Dried Fruit Compote 34
Dutch Baby Pancake 105

E
Eggplant, Stuffed 39

F
Fajitas 118
Family Potluck Chicken 116
Family Vegetable Soup 122
Frittata, Vegetable 124
Fruit Chutney 102
Fruit, Dried Compote 34

G
Gazpacho 63
Giant Dutch Baby Pancake 105
Graham Bread 95
Grilled Lemon Chicken 70
Grilled Marinated Salmon 78

H
Happy Spices Sauce 27
Harvest Vegetable Basket 94
Hearty Peasant Bread 37
Hot Apricot Souffle 44
Hot Potato Salad 79
Hummus Spread 113

J
Jennifer's Angel Food Cake 91

L
Lamb Roasted in Parchment 31
Lemon Chicken, Grilled 70
Lemon Rice and Zucchini Pilaf 120
Lemon Slush 50
Light Mayonnaise 114

M
Mango Puree 45
Marcelle's Pesto Mousse 112
Marinated Salmon 78
Marinated Vegetable Platter 83
Mayonnaise, Light 114
Melon and Raspberries in Galliano 85
Melon Soup, Chilled 20
Mexican Rice, Williams 119
Middle Eastern Chicken 126
Mint Tea 34
Mocha Sabayon 61
Muffins, Apple Carrot Bran 107

O
Oatmeal Hearts 28
Oranges in Sangria 73
Oranges with Fennel and Red Onion 100
Oriental Chicken Salad 21
Oriental Noodle Salad 26
Osso Buco 84

P
Pancake, Giant Dutch Baby 105
Papillote of Seafood 59
Pasta
  Angel Hair with Crab etc. 43
  Pesto Sauce for pasta 112
  Spinach Pinwheels 48
Pea Pods, Stuffed with Scallops and Shrimps 52
Peach Chutney 102
Peppers, Stuffed Red and Green 38
Pesto Mousse 112
Pineapple-Orange Sorbet 103
Pizza
  Crust 88
  Primavera 89
  Prosciutto and Cantaloupe 90
  Seafood 89
  Smoked Salmon 90
  Tomato Sauce for Pizza 89
Poached Pears 80
Pommes Parisienne 65
Porridge-on-the-Run 130
Potato Salad, Hot 79
Prawn and Chicken Curry 101
Prawns with Tropical Dip 75
Primavera Salad 25
Puree of Carrots and Yams 66

R
Rabbit Stew with Eggplant 121
Raisins in Port 102
Raspberry Puree 22
Raspberry Sauce 81
Ratatouille 125
Red Pepper Oil 26
Red Pepper-Yogurt Mousse 111
Red Snapper with Peppers 123
Rice, Basmati 102
Rice Bulgar Pilaf 72
Rice, Lemon Brown and Zucchini Pilaf 120
Rice Pudding, Spanish 129
Risotto 54
Roast Lamb in Parchment 31

S
Salad Dressings
  Basil Vinaigrette 42
  Green Peppercorn Dressing 71
  Shallot Vinaigrette 24
  Yogurt Dressing 114
Salads
  Hot Potato Salad 79
  Oranges with Fennel and Red Onions 100
  Oriental Chicken Salad 21
  Oriental Noodle Salad 25
  Primavera Salad 24
  Spinach Salad with Chevre 76
  Tomato Salad 42
  Walnut-Blue Cheese Salad 58
Salmon Grilled with Onions 78
Salmon Tartare 69
Salsa 93
Sauces
  Apple Sauce 106
  Creme Anglaise 80
  Curry Sauce 25
  Happy Spices Sauce 27
  Mango Puree 45
  Mocha Sabayon 61
  Pesto Sauce 112
  Raspberry Puree 22
  Raspberry Sauce 81
  Salsa 93
  Tomato Coulis 108
  Tropical Dip 75
Scallopine, Veal 53
Seafood
  Pasta with Crab etc. 43
  Prawn and Chicken Curry 101
  Prawns with Tropical Dip 75

Red Snapper with Peppers 123
Salmon, Grilled with Onions 78
Salmon Tartare 69
Scallops and Shrimp-Stuffed Pea Pods 52
Seafood Papillote 59
Seafood Pizza 89
Shrimp and Scallop Seviche 110
Stuffed Sole with Citrus 64
Seviche, Shrimp and Scallop 110
Shallot Vinaigrette 25
Shredded Zucchini and Carrot Saute 72
Smoked Salmon Pizza 90
Sole, Stuffed with Shrimp and Citrus 64
Soups
Apple Mulled Wine Soup 87
Black Bean Soup 96
Chilled Cucumber-Yogurt Soup 36
Chilled Melon Soup 20
Family Vegetable Soup 122
Gazpacho 63
Strawberries 'n Champagne Soup 105
Zucchini-Dill Soup 30
Spanish Rice Pudding 129
Spiced Coffee 34
Spinach Pinwheels 48
Spinach Salad with Chevre 76
Spinach Stuffing, for Turkey Breast 24
Spritzer 20
Steamed Prawns 75
Strawberries 'n Champagne Soup 105
Strawberry-Banana Freeze 130
Strawberry Goblets, Shimmering 40
Stuffed Eggplant 39
Stuffed Pea Pods 52
Stuffed Peppers 38
Stuffed Tomatoes 115
Stuffed Zucchini 40

T
Tomato Coulis 108
Tomato Salad 42
Tomato Sauce for Pizza 89
Tomatoes, Stuffed 115
Tomato-Zucchini Medley 55
Tropical Dip 75
Tropical Mousse 56
Turkey Breast with Spinach Stuffing 24

V
Veal Scallopine with Lemon 53
Vegetable Basket, Yogurt Dip 94
Vegetable Casserole 32
Vegetable Curry 117
Vegetable Frittata 124
Vegetable Platter, Marinated 83
Vegetable Soup, Family's 122

W
Walnut-Blue Cheese Salad 58
Wholewheat Bagel Crisps 77
Williams Mexican Rice 119

Y
Yogurt Coffee Cake 127
Yogurt Dip 94
Yogurt Salad Dressing 114

Z
Zucchini and Carrot Saute 72
Zucchini Dill Soup 30
Zucchini, Stuffed 40
Zucchini-Tomato Medley 55